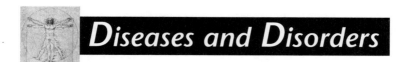

# SARS

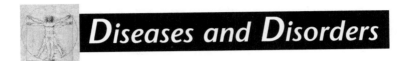

# SARS

Titles in the Diseases and Disorders series include:

Acne
Alzheimer's Disease
Anthrax
Anorexia and Bulimia
Arthritis
Asthma
Attention Deficit Disorder
Autism
Breast Cancer
Cerebral Palsy
Chronic Fatigue Syndrome
Cystic Fibrosis
Diabetes
Down Syndrome
Epilepsy
Headaches
Hemophilia
Hepatitis
Learning Disabilities
Leukemia
Lyme Disease
Multiple Sclerosis
Obesity
Phobias
Schizophrenia
Sexually Transmitted Diseases
Sleep Disorders
Smallpox
West Nile Virus

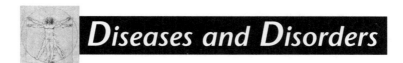
*Diseases and Disorders*

# SARS

Gail B. Stewart

LUCENT
BOOKS®

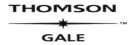
THOMSON
™
GALE

San Diego • Detroit • New York • San Francisco • Cleveland
New Haven, Conn. • Waterville, Maine • London • Munich

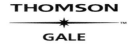

**THOMSON**

**GALE**

© 2004 by Lucent Books. Lucent Books is an imprint of The Gale Group, Inc., a division of Thomson Learning, Inc.

Lucent Books® and Thomson Learning™ are trademarks used herein under license.

*For more information, contact*
Lucent Books
27500 Drake Rd.
Farmington Hills, MI 48331-3535
Or you can visit our Internet site at www.gale.com

**LIBRARY OF CONGRESS CATALOGING-IN-PUBLICATION DATA**

Stewart, Gail, B.
  SARS/ by Gail B. Stewart.
    v. cm. — (Diseases and disorders series)
Includes bibliographical references and index.
Summary: Describes SARS, its effects on the world's economy, treatments for the disease, and what may happen if it was to return.
Contents: The Secret Killer—Investigating SARS—SARS, Politics, and the Economy—Life with SARS—SARS and the Future.
  ISBN 1-59018-529-3 (hardback : alk. paper)
  I. Title. II. Series.

Printed in the United States of America

# *Table of Contents*

Foreword                                          8

Introduction
   The Faces of SARS                         10

Chapter 1
   The Secret Killer                         13

Chapter 2
   Investigating SARS                        28

Chapter 3
   Life with SARS                            44

Chapter 4
   SARS, Politics, and the Economy           60

Chapter 5
   SARS and the Future                       76

   Notes                                     91
   Organizations to Contact                  97
   For Further Reading                       99
   Works Consulted                          101
   Index                                    105
   Picture Credits                          111
   About the Author                         112

# "The Most Difficult Puzzles Ever Devised"

CHARLES BEST, ONE of the pioneers in the search for a cure for diabetes, once explained what it is about medical research that intrigued him so. "It's not just the gratification of knowing one is helping people," he confided, "although that probably is a more heroic and selfless motivation. Those feelings may enter in, but truly, what I find best is the feeling of going toe to toe with nature, of trying to solve the most difficult puzzles ever devised. The answers are there somewhere, those keys that will solve the puzzle and make the patient well. But how will those keys be found?"

Since the dawn of civilization, nothing has so puzzled people—and often frightened them, as well—as the onset of illness in a body or mind that had seemed healthy before. A seizure, the inability of a heart to pump, the sudden deterioration of muscle tone in a small child—being unable to reverse such conditions or even to understand why they occur was unspeakably frustrating to healers. Even before there were names for such conditions, even before they were understood at all, each was a reminder of how complex the human body was, and how vulnerable.

While our grappling with understanding diseases has been frustrating at times, it has also provided some of humankind's most heroic accomplishments. Alexander Fleming's accidental discovery in 1928 of a mold that could be turned into penicillin has resulted in the saving of untold millions of lives. The isolation of the enzyme insulin has reversed what was once a death sentence for anyone with diabetes. There have been great strides in combating conditions for which there is not yet a cure, too. Medicines can help AIDS patients live longer, diagnostic tools such as mammography and ultrasounds can help doctors find tumors while they are treatable, and laser surgery techniques have made the most intricate, minute operations routine.

This "toe-to-toe" competition with diseases and disorders is even more remarkable when seen in a historical continuum. An astonishing amount of progress has been made in a very short time. Just two hundred years ago, the existence of germs as a cause of some diseases was unknown. In fact, it was less than 150 years ago that a British surgeon named Joseph Lister had difficulty persuading his fellow doctors that washing their hands before delivering a baby might increase the chances of a healthy delivery (especially if they had just attended to a diseased patient)!

Each book in Lucent's Diseases and Disorders series explores a disease or disorder and the knowledge that has been accumulated (or discarded) by doctors through the years. Each book also examines the tools used for pinpointing a diagnosis, as well as the various means that are used to treat or cure a disease. Finally, new ideas are presented—techniques or medicines that may be on the horizon.

Frustration and disappointment are still part of medicine, for not every disease or condition can be cured or prevented. But the limitations of knowledge are being pushed outward constantly; the "most difficult puzzles ever devised" are finding challengers every day.

# The Faces of SARS

IT SEEMED, IN the early months of 2003, that the disease came out of nowhere. No one could pinpoint the first case of severe acute respiratory syndrome (SARS)—it probably occurred in November 2002—but by early 2003 it was roaring through hospitals in China and other parts of Asia, as well as in Toronto, Canada, striking down hundreds of doctors and nurses as they tried to care for their patients. It was a ghastly illness; one Hong Kong resident says that watching someone with SARS gasp and fight for breath was "like watching a man drown to death on dry land."[1]

Thousands of those infected died, and doctors were panicking, for there seemed to be little progress in fighting the new disease, and it continued to spread. As people quickly learned, a dangerous new disease in the age of jet travel rapidly becomes everyone's problem. By June 2003 there were SARS victims on six continents.

## Many Effects

Of course, those primarily affected by the disease were people who became infected with SARS. Henry Likyuen Chan, a thirty-four-year-old doctor in Hong Kong, contracted SARS in the hospital where he works. His high fever and racking cough led his doctors to fear the worst. In fact, one colleague cried when she heard Chan's gasping attempts to breathe. He eventually recovered, but it is clear that the battle with SARS was the most difficult thing he had ever encountered. "I am quite an aggressive person," he says. "That is why I was determined to conquer SARS."[2]

But the effects of SARS have been felt by more than the patients and their families. In hundreds of smaller ways, people all over the world had their routines altered because of the disease. Students who had planned on studying in China were told by the Centers for Disease Control to cancel their plans. One twenty-one-year-old law student from Virginia had just begun an internship in Hong Kong when the outbreak hit, and he was called home.

In SARS-affected regions, businesses that rely on travelers and tourists struggled and were often forced to cut their work force to meet payrolls. Airlines with flights to Hong Kong and mainland China were especially hard-hit. In Toronto a girls' soccer team had won the right to compete in an exhibition match in Pennsylvania, but the team's coach was told not to come after all. One of the players, a sixteen-year-old, had hoped to show her skills and perhaps get a college scholarship. "It was my one big chance," she says. "I was literally crushed."[3]

*At a 2003 Toronto Bluejays baseball game, a man wears a surgical mask to protect himself from the SARS virus.*

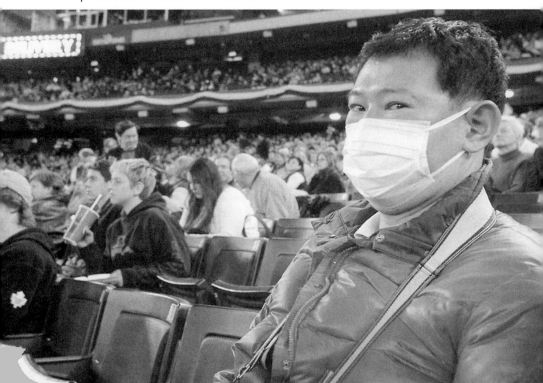

Lily, a sixteen-year-old ice skater from St. Paul, Minnesota, had been planning to attend a clinic in Toronto in April 2003. However, when SARS began spreading in that city, health officials urged travelers to postpone visits until later. "But the clinic isn't offered later," she says. "It was my chance to work with a really good coach, and it couldn't happen. My mom says I should have more perspective about this, and think about people who have SARS and are suffering. I know she's right; they've got it worse off than me, but I'm still really disappointed."[4]

## Unsettling Questions

The emergence of SARS and its spread throughout the world has raised unsettling questions about contagious disease and medicine's ability to prevent it. More than ever before, researchers are eager to understand how viruses arise. How can they mutate, and why do some viruses cause so much damage to the human body, while others have only faint effects?

While some strides have been made in understanding the nature of the SARS virus, a great deal is left unanswered. In a world that has recently begun to consider bioterrorism a very possible threat, the SARS virus has demonstrated how vulnerable life is in the face of a new and contagious disease, and how societies, governments, and economies can be rattled by the tiniest of microbes.

# Chapter 1

# The Secret Killer

MONTHS BEFORE THE World Health Organization declared it a worldwide health threat and gave the disease its name, SARS had begun infecting people in Guangdong Province, in southern China. At the beginning, however, few health professionals were worried about it at all.

## A Cold? The Flu?

It was in November 2002 that the first cases were seen in the rural areas of Guangdong Province. People complained about headaches, aching muscles and joints, as well as a loss of appetite. Few sufferers were concerned; it was November, after all, and it was not unusual to catch a cold or flu during the cool, rainy season. Most continued going to work or school, believing that the symptoms would fade after a few days.

Within three or four days, however, patients found that they felt worse, not better. Many were experiencing dry coughs, fever, and difficulty breathing. Doctors believed it was pneumonia, and prescribed antibiotics and rest. But this disease did not respond to antibiotics or any of the usual remedies for pneumonia. Some patients developed such difficulty breathing that they were hooked up to respirators. Others died, blue-faced and gasping futilely for breath, even with the respirators.

As the weeks passed, doctors in the local Guangdong hospitals believed that they were dealing with a very different sort of pneumonia than they had ever seen before. The worst part was that, unlike typical pneumonia, this disease appeared to be highly contagious. The first patients who sought help from local hospitals left a trail of infected health care workers in their wake as they sought relief from their labored breathing and high fevers.

## "We Didn't Take Any Preventive Measures"

One young nurse who became ill says that she had been looking after a patient who came to the hospital with flu-like symptoms, as well as a severe cough. "The whole forty minutes [she was with him] he was coughing and expelling huge amounts of phlegm." This was unusual, she says, for a cough of that nature was not normally a symptom of the strains of flu she had seen. But although his illness was a mystery, the staff did not wear masks when tending to him. "We didn't take any preventive measures," she says, "as we normally don't wear masks when taking care of flu patients."[5]

The patient's condition deteriorated quickly, and he was transferred to a larger urban hospital, where he died. Meanwhile, the nurse became ill. With a high fever, aches, and fatigue, she thought she might be overworked or had maybe caught the flu.

*A doctor treats a SARS patient in Hanoi, Vietnam, in 2003. The first cases of the disease appeared in November 2002 in rural areas of China's Guangdong Province.*

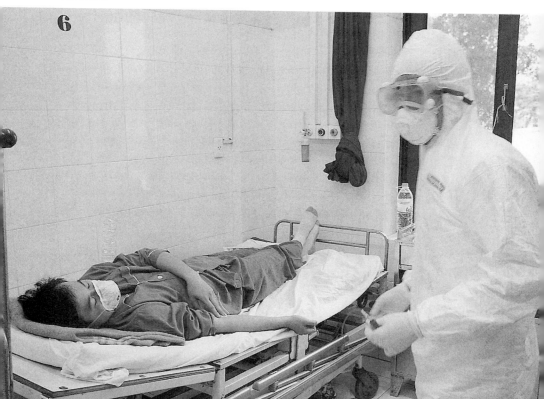

But medicines and rest did not help her symptoms at all, and she was admitted to the hospital where ten other staff members had become sick with similar complaints.

Her symptoms worsened within a day or two. "Breathing was difficult and I had to be under a respirator for about ten days. I was unconscious most of the time." Though she was lucky enough to survive, after more than a month she was still ill:

> My lungs haven't got back to normal and I still feel tight in the chest. I suffer from a bad insomnia; most nights I can only sleep for a couple hours. My muscles are so weak I can hardly lift anything, and my eyes are swollen and red. But the thing that disturbs me the most is my right leg. I can't walk, can't even move the leg without feeling an excruciating pain in my joints. I used to be very active, very physical.[6]

## News via the Grapevine

But even though there were many such stories among people who were battling the disease, the Chinese remained secretive. They refused to release information about the illness in the newspapers or television. Government officials did not want to alarm the citizens, nor did they want to admit that there was a contagious, deadly disease that they were unable to contain. Such an admission would cause a mass panic and would almost certainly affect the foreign investment on which China had become dependent. Since the Chinese media are all tightly controlled by the government, no details were released about the disease, and doctors were told not to discuss it—even with health professionals in other parts of China.

However, many Chinese health care workers were alarmed by the disease, and on many of the most popular Chinese Internet sites doctors and nurses passed along rumors that people were dying from a mysterious new form of pneumonia. It soon became clear to provincial officials that they could not remain silent about the disease. On February 11, 2003, Guangdong officials ordered the health minister to make a public announcement, acknowledging that there was a form of pneumonia that had killed

*In an effort to prevent widespread panic, Chinese government officials refused to release information to the press about the new disease.*

five people and infected hundreds of others. At the same time, however, the health minister reassured the Chinese people that there was nothing to fear, since the disease was now completely under control.

The government in Beijing, China's capital, was worried about the effects of such news on China's reputation as a modern, growing nation. Determined that there be no further rumors or questions about the disease, officials ordered the people of Guangdong to refrain from talking about it. It was best, they warned, "to voluntarily uphold social stability, not believe in rumors, not spread rumors."[7] In addition, the police were instructed to meet with Chinese Internet webmasters and order them to write only positive things on their websites about the nation's efforts to combat the disease.

## Coming to the City

But it was difficult for the people in Guangdong to remain silent about SARS when it was obvious that the disease was not under control at all. In fact, there was a growing problem as some rural patients—frightened because they were not getting better in their local hospitals—traveled to Guangzhou, the large capital city of the province. Because of the lack of information on the disease, the large metropolitan hospitals of Guangzhou were unaware of the seriousness and highly contagious nature of SARS. While the local hospitals had learned to isolate SARS patients to keep them from infecting others, the metropolitcan hospitals found out the hard way.

Nurses at the Number 2 People's Hospital in Guangzhou say that they will always remember February 2003 as a time when they were all endangered. A very sick man had visited various hospitals in the city—including Number 2. No health care workers

*A Hong Kong shopkeeper prepares an herbal remedy for a SARS patient. Many Chinese turned to folk remedies to protect themselves from the disease.*

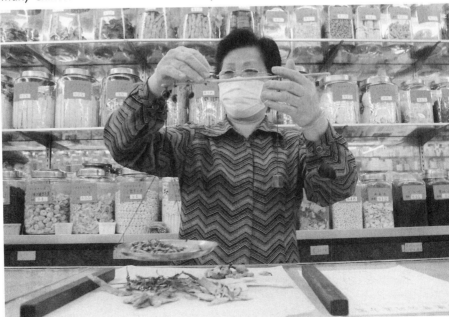

knew enough about SARS to isolate the man; in fact, none of the staff who examined him used masks or gloves. As a result, dozens of doctors and nurses became infected. Says one nurse from Number 2, "He was very sick, but who knew there was something so terrible going around?"[8]

The rapid growth of the number of cases began to cause panic among the public in Guangdong. "On the streets here," noted *New York Times* reporter Elizabeth Rosenthal who was visiting Guangdong Province, "rumors abound, and people feel they cannot protect themselves in the absence of information."[9] That absence of information left a vacuum that was quickly filled by various theories about the nature of the disease, ranging from an exotic form of flu to anthrax or some other weapon that had leaked from a military base. Hoping to protect themselves from the germs, people wore surgical masks on the streets, and if they could not find the real thing, they fashioned them from gauze and tape.

A number of folk remedies were circulated, too—from breathing vinegar fumes to eating a diet of turnips. One cure, adopted by many frightened Chinese, was to smoke more cigarettes—or, if one did not already smoke, then start. Advocates of this cure believed that the tobacco smoke would drive the poisons from patients' lungs, allowing them to breathe more easily. But neither the folk remedies nor the antibiotics were effective against SARS, and Chinese health officials were worried.

## "We Didn't Believe It"

Though Chinese officials had tried to keep SARS a secret, bits and pieces of information about the disease had spread via the Internet to the World Health Organization (WHO) and the Centers for Disease Control (CDC)—both international public health organizations. When WHO's Outbreak Center, which investigates any new and potentially hazardous diseases in the world, made official inquiries to China, they were told that the oubreak was a new type of flu—and that the Chinese health authorities could handle it without outside help.

But as word of a growing death count continued to reach beyond China's borders, WHO and CDC officials were convinced that they were being lied to. Chinese officials refused to provide more specific information and repeated orders to its doctors not to respond to any inquiries from WHO or the CDC. Certain that there must be more going on in China, WHO officials contacted a Hong Kong laboratory with which they frequently worked, and had lab technicians visit Guangdong hospitals to collect tissue samples from some patients.

Worried about losing their jobs, however, the Chinese health officials provided tissue samples from patients who were suffering from other germs, and repeated that the outbreak was over. Doctors at the international agencies were skeptical, since antibiotics would certainly have cured all of the germs in those samples. One CDC doctor said flatly, "We didn't believe it."[10] As he would learn very soon, his instincts were absolutely correct.

## Spreading Beyond Guangdong's Borders

On February 21, 2003, the one thing that was feared most occurred—SARS spread beyond Guangdong Province's borders. A sixty-four-year-old retired lung specialist from Guangdong named Liu Jianlun went to Hong Kong for his nephew's wedding. Liu had been feeling tired, and when he arrived in Hong Kong he was running a low-grade fever.

As Liu's symptoms worsened, he went to a Hong Kong hospital. Understanding that he probably had SARS, Liu advised the emergency room staff to isolate him behind double panes of glass, which Guangdong regional hospitals had begun doing for their patients. He also insisted that before examining him, doctors and nurses put on protective masks, gloves, and gowns. Liu's cautions undoubtedly saved lives at the hospital; he died several days later, but none of the staff became infected.

But Liu's death was not publicized, nor were doctors in other hospitals in Hong Kong or other places told about the incident. And because he was contagious before he went to the hospital, he inadvertently infected a number of people at the same hotel where he was staying. Three young women from Singapore were infected, as were two Canadians, a man from Hong Kong, and an American businessman on his way to Hanoi, Vietnam. Not only had SARS been carried beyond the borders of Guangdong, China, but because of this one case, it would soon be spread throughout the world.

## A Global Threat

Again, because of the lack of real information about the disease, hospitals outside of Guangdong Province were ill-equipped to deal with it. In Toronto, for example, a woman who had talked to Liu in Hong Kong became ill and died on March 5, 2003, after infecting her son and several doctors and nurses at the Toronto hospital where she was taken.

When her son Tse visited the emergency room of the same hospital on March 7, staff doctors and nurses knew nothing about the disease and had no idea how contagious Tse was. "He had a fever and a cough," remembers one nurse, "and he was having a hard time catching his breath. And he looked scared."[11]

Tse was placed in a bed of an observation ward and infected two men in nearby beds, who in the days ahead infected dozens of others with whom they had contact. "At that point," says one Toronto doctor, "there was no concept of how infectious [Tse] was."[12] By May 15 there would be at least 145 cases of SARS, with nineteen people dead of the disease.

## An Official Alert

With new information that the disease had spread to Canada and other countries, WHO officials issued a global alert on March 12, 2003. With the limited amount of information it possessed, the agency warned of the new disease and urged travelers and airline crews around the world to watch for symptoms. It also recommended that doctors and nurses isolate anyone presenting symptoms that seemed suspicious and take precautions by using protective suits, gloves, and masks when treating patients.

The warning to health professionals was apt, for doctors and nurses were among the hardest hit by SARS. By the middle of March 2003 the emergency room at Scarborough Grace Hospital, where Tse was treated, had to shut down because of a shortage of healthy staff members. Thousands of Toronto citizens who had visited the hospital or had been treated there were told to isolate themselves at home for ten days to avoid infecting others.

In Hanoi, the American businessman infected twenty health care workers. Of the three women from Singapore, one visited the Tan Tock Seng Hospital, and left ninety-two people sick—at least one-third of them health care workers.

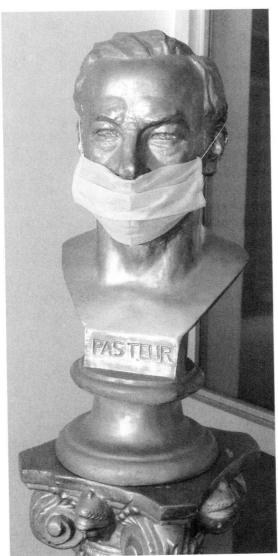

*At the entrance to a hospital in Hanoi, Vietnam, a bust of French chemist Louis Pasteur wears a surgical mask. From China, SARS quickly spread into neighboring Vietnam.*

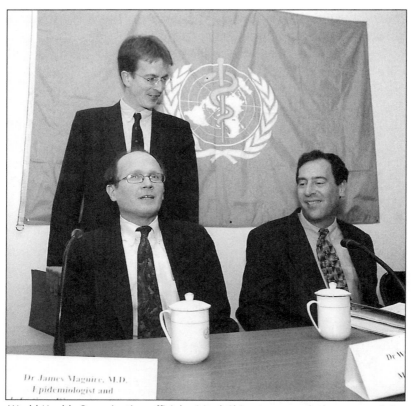

*World Health Organization officials visited China to research the extent of the SARS outbreak. Initially, the Chinese government refused to cooperate with the officials.*

## Worst in China

China remained the hardest hit by the growing epidemic, and the government continued its policy of secrecy and noncooperation with international authorities. WHO asked for permission to visit China so that doctors could review data about the first outbreak in Guangdong. The response by the Chinese was, says one WHO official, "dead silence."[13]

The fact that their government was continuing to be secretive caused panic among the Chinese public. Villages erected barriers on the roads leading in and out of town to be sure that outsiders did not bring the disease in. Rumors circulated like wildfire, too, noted one observer. "Grannies . . . whispered that the entire capital was going to be quarantined, while Internet chat rooms buzzed with claims that the disease was a conspiracy courtesy of the Americans and the Taiwanese."[14]

In early April SARS hit Beijing, infecting ninety people at a large downtown hospital—seventy of them nurses and doctors. Yet when asked if it was safe for tourists to come to the city, one government representative minimized the risks, stating that there had been only thirty-seven cases, and the disease had been contained by Chinese health care workers. "Of course [tourists] can travel," he said. "We think it's very safe."[15]

## "We're Frustrated"

International health officials, however, were not convinced. One WHO representative was adamant that the stonewalling had to stop. "We have clearly told the government," he said, "the international community doesn't trust your figures."[16] Many doctors around the world demanded more information in case SARS appeared among their citizens. In the United States, Secretary of Health and Human Services Tommy Thompson also expressed his exasperation with the Chinese government for being overly concerned about their image and insisted that WHO and the CDC only wanted to help China contain the disease. "We're frustrated," he said. "We want to work in greater collaboration with them."[17]

By the end of April, however, the government finally acknowledged that SARS was not completely contained and that an accurate count of those with SARS in Beijing was 339, rather than 37, as previously announced. Within a week, the figure had jumped to 900 confirmed cases. To try to contain the disease, the government ordered the quarantine of all offices, hotels, restaurants, and residential buildings that might have been visited by people infected with SARS. By quarantining, or isolating, people who were already sick or who had been exposed to the disease, doctors hoped to minimize the chance of them infecting more people. The order for a two-week quarantine left more than two thousand doctors, nurses, and patients at Peking University's

People's Hospital in downtown Beijing isolated among 90 confirmed cases of SARS—70 of them health care workers.

Although the government stressed that there was little to fear, Beijing residents were behaving otherwise. By the end of the month the city of 13 million resembled a ghost town, most citizens having taken refuge in their homes, hoping to avoid catching the disease that the government refused to talk about openly.

While these were aggressive steps for Chinese leaders to take, many experts believe that the government was still attempting to hide the extent of the epidemic from WHO and the rest of the world. For instance, China's leaders were so worried about an outbreak in Shanghai, the nation's banking and commercial center, that they ordered Shanghai officials to preserve the city's reputation as "SARS-free" at any cost. Doctors in Shanghai, however, admitted to reporters that there were at least 30 con-

*A World Health Organization official meets with reporters after the Chinese government allowed him to examine patients afflicted with SARS.*

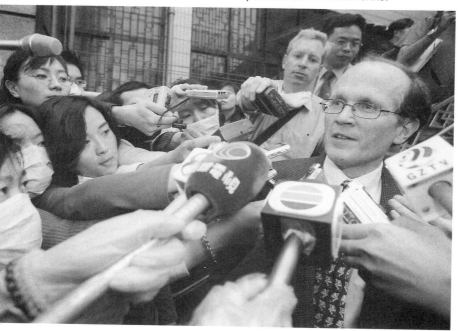

firmed cases in the city already, but the government was firm in its order. "All I have been told," one health official in Shanghai explains, "is that we must maintain the image of Shanghai as a place without a SARS problem."[18]

## Hiding in Ambulances

Even when WHO representatives were finally permitted to enter China for the purpose of investigating the nature of the disease, the stonewalling continued. Chinese doctors were instructed to follow what was called the policy of the "Three No's"—"No talking to the media about the nature of SARS; no talking to the public about doctors' personal experiences treating the disease; and no communicating with the WHO about anything to do with SARS."[19]

When WHO representatives visited Beijing's China-Japan Friendship Hospital on April 21, 2003, for example, they were shown a ward containing only two SARS patients. The rest, says reporter Hannah Beech, were being driven around the city in ambulances until the WHO doctors left the hospital. "Inside the ambulances," she explains, "was a deadly secret: 31 coughing, shivering hospital Workers who had caught . . . SARS from their patients."[20]

Fearing that they would be fired if they talked to the international media, doctors and nurses remained silent when asked about the epidemic. Their only comments were off the record, and at those times they admitted that the threat of SARS throughout the country was far more than the government was letting on. One doctor apologized that he was not allowed to speak with an American reporter. "I'm embarrassed that I can't talk to you," he said. "I had really wanted to, but I'm young, and I can't afford to lose my job."[21]

One health minister, however, was angry that China was being judged harshly by other nations for its methods of dealing with the crisis. He feels that because China is such a populous nation, the government cannot afford to make decisions based on what is best for individual people, but rather must think of the majority. "You foreigners value each person's life more than we do because you

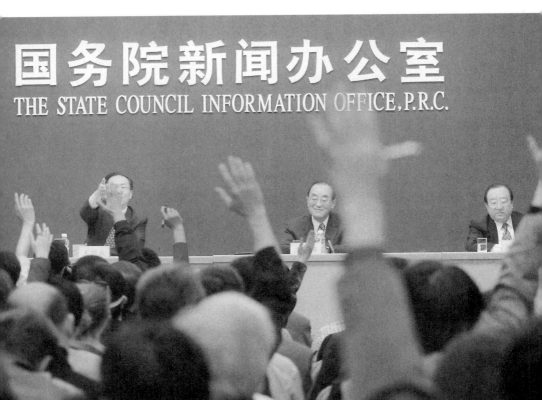

*Chinese government officials brief reporters about the SARS virus in April 2003 after 250 residents of a Hong Kong apartment complex contracted the disease.*

have fewer people in your countries," he says. "Our primary concern is social stability, and if a few people's deaths are kept secret, it's worth it to keep things stable."[22]

## More Questions than Answers

But stability was hard to maintain as the disease continued to spread. Doctors had believed that SARS was spread only by close human contact—from inhaling the spray of a cough or sneeze of an infected person. In Hong Kong, however, that theory proved false. In less than a week, 250 residents of a thirty-three-floor housing development contracted SARS, and most of those people had never met one another. Clearly, close human contact had not occurred, yet the disease spread quickly—by the end of April infecting a total of 1,527 in Hong Kong.

As in other cities around the world, quarantine seemed the only method of containing SARS, although doctors were not even certain whether that would work. Meanwhile, hospitals were running out of space, people were fleeing affected areas, and those who had been exposed to the disease were herded into seclusion until doctors felt that they were no longer at risk of coming down with SARS.

As doctors and researchers struggled for answers, they were met with more questions. Where did the disease come from, and how exactly was it spread? Was there any medication that would help SARS victims? One Toronto doctor voiced his frustration as more patients with symptoms continued to show up in the city's emergency rooms. "The difficulty is we're facing an enemy that has no known shape, no identity, and no known effective treatment—and that's causing the most concern."[23] Clearly, the international medical community had a difficult task ahead.

# Chapter 2

# Investigating SARS

L ONG BEFORE SARS was an international epidemic—when it was still a mysterious disease affecting people in Guangdong Province, doctors around the world were hearing rumors by way of the Internet. Always concerned about the emersion of a new illness, WHO researchers around the world were keeping track of any information they could get about the pneumonia-type illness.

## Six Percent

Any new disease causes worry, and there have been a number of killers that have emerged in the past quarter century—from AIDS to Ebola. In addition, WHO doctors around the world have monitored oubreaks of well-known but dangerous diseases such as malaria and cholera. In many cases, the disease can be identified and contained in one area before it spreads out of control. However, the most frightening of all scenarios, say experts, is that a highly contagious disease that is unknown to doctors reaches an international airport, thus spreading it to other nations before anyone is even aware of it. That is just what happened with SARS.

Of course, no one knew then how deadly the disease might be or how contagious. The numbers of people dying of SARS were very small compared with, say, the numbers dying from AIDS in a single year—which totaled 3 million worldwide in 2002. With the data they had, doctors estimated that the death rate of SARS was about 6 percent—in other words, of every one hundred people infected with SARS, six died.

Six percent is a fairly low death rate as long as the disease is relatively contained in a particular area and not extremely contagious. However, with a disease that spreads easily from person to person, it is an extremely worrisome rate. Researchers point to a strain of flu in 1918 with a death rate of less than three percent, but which was so highly contagious that it killed between 25 million and 40 million people worldwide in eighteen months.

As time went on and more people became infected with SARS, doctors became more alarmed. One aspect of the new disease that worried WHO researchers was the high infection rate among health professionals. In Hanoi, Vietnam, for example, 56 percent of the doctors and nurses who came into contact with the disease became infected. Says Julie Gerberding, director of the CDC, "We never see that kind of rate."[24]

WHO officials alerted the CDC in Atlanta, informing them that as soon as WHO doctors were able to get tissue and blood samples from patients with the disease, they would send them to

*Patients in Singapore wait to be tested for SARS. Although SARS has a relatively low death rate, the disease is particularly worrisome because of its highly contagious nature.*

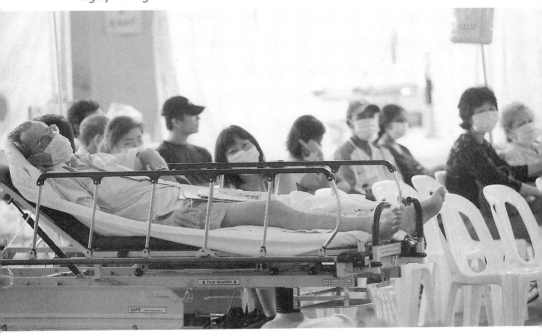

the CDC's Building 15, where the most feared diseases on the planet are studied. From what doctors knew about SARS thus far, it seemed to fit in the category of what are known as special pathogens—germs that are both contagious and deadly, with the potential to kill a great many victims.

## Guessing Wrong

Tissue and blood specimens were delayed, however. For one thing, autopsies are quite rare in most Asian hospitals, and doctors at first were reluctant to authorize the taking of lung tissue samples. When some hospitals were finally persuaded to begin releasing specimens, their transport to the research facilities was delayed because many international shippers refused to carry

*Because they have weak immune systems, ducks are breeding grounds for new viruses. Many disease-causing viruses originate with animals.*

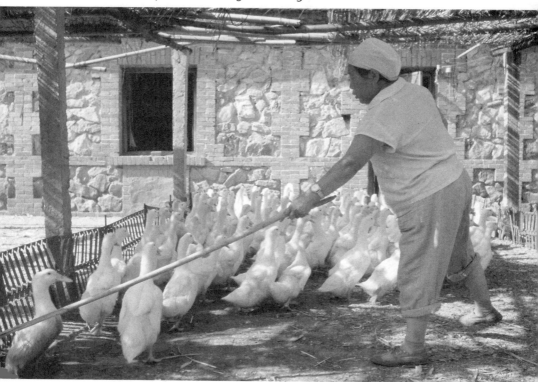

such hazardous material. By March 10, 2003, specimens were brought to various research facilities—including Building 15 in Atlanta—by U.S. military planes, and doctors began to inspect the vials of blood, sputum, and bits of tissue from patients' lungs or throats.

One of the early assumptions about SARS was that it would prove to be a new type of influenza, or flu virus. After all, many strains of flu have originated in rural areas of China, where people and livestock often live very close to one another. Epidemiologists, doctors who study the transmission of diseases, say that many viruses that cause disease in humans actually originate with animals. Ducks, because they have weak immune systems, seem to be breeding grounds for new viruses. In a duck's body, such viruses can mutate and then are able to jump to pigs, and from pigs to people. Many strains of flu have originated this way in southern China, where the living conditions of ducks, pigs, and people create what one researcher termed "a toxic stew."[25]

Other news gave researchers even more support for their theory of a new strain of flu. They heard of a new bird flu in China that had made some people sick. Perhaps, doctors reasoned, the strange new SARS disease was another mutation of the bird virus, but this time more virulent and contagious than usual. "We put one and one together," explains one researcher, "and thought this was the [bird flu virus] beginning its trip around the world."[26]

## A Difficult Job for a Crisis Team

The scramble to learn about the mystery disease began in mid-March, when WHO doctors were alerted that a Toronto woman had become infected. Apparently, SARS had hopped continents. WHO issued its first global warning, alerting travelers that what appeared to be a very dangerous contagious disease had become a worldwide health threat.

On March 17, 2003, WHO officials called the top epidemiologists throughout the world to form a crisis team that would tackle the problem of identifying the cause of the disease. Doctors in China had easily ruled out bacteria as the cause of SARS.

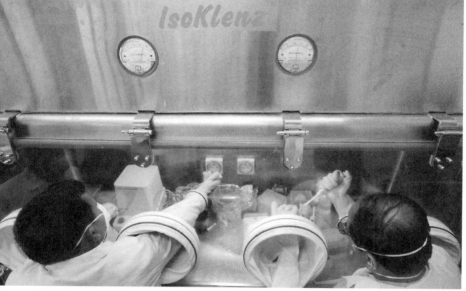

*Researchers were able to deduce that a virus is responsible for SARS because the pathogen did not respond to antibiotics and was invisible under a microscope.*

Bacteria would have been visible under their microscopes, and antibiotics, which are powerful killers of bacteria, would have had an effect on the disease. The prevailing theory was that it was a virus, but even for the best researchers in the world, identifying the virus would be difficult. After all, it had taken more than three years for researchers to isolate and identify the AIDS virus.

Identifying viruses is far more difficult than identifying bacteria. Bacteria are living organisms and can be observed with a fairly standard microscope. Viruses, however, are very tiny—some are a million times smaller than bacteria. In addition, viruses act in different ways than bacteria, since they can survive only when inside a living cell. In fact, scientists believe that viruses are not true living things, since they cannot survive or reproduce on their own. Seeing and identifying one extremely tiny virus within a cell, when scientists are not aware of what they are looking for, is difficult, time-consuming work.

## "The Medical Equivalent of Shock and Awe"

There are other factors that often slow work for scientists. Laboratories are exceptionally expensive places to run, and scientists are often in competition with one another to find a new medicine or vaccine that can bring in funds for research. For that reason, research facilities are rarely willing to consolidate or share information, since they view one another as rivals. And because there is no greater achievement for a scientist than discovering a pathogen or its cure, the scientists themselves are often competitors.

The director of WHO's crisis team, Dr. Klaus Stohr, says that because of the immediate threat of the new disease, it was not difficult to convince the doctors to lay aside the competitiveness. They agreed to work together, sharing patient data, lab results, and other information. "These are all famous microbiologists whose life's dream is to discover a virus, put their name on it and win the Nobel Prize," says Stohr. "But they understand that our only chance to put this thing back in the bottle is if we all work together."[27]

Stohr set up a website with a secure password for the participating epidemiologists. He also arranged twice-a-day conference calls so the team could discuss any new theories or ideas, results of lab tests, and so on. The results were beyond anything Stohr could have anticipated. Not only did the team identify the cause of the disease, but it did so in less than seven weeks. The speed at which the battle against SARS was waged, says one researcher, was "the medical equivalent of shock and awe [the phrase President George W. Bush had used to describe the U.S. attack on Baghdad in March 2003]."[28]

## A Surprising Culprit

The first significant step in the process was to drop infected tissue or blood into flasks of cells containing a culture of monkey kidney cells, called Vero cells. Vero cells are especially good for breeding viruses, and scientists often use a Vero cell solution to indicate the presence of a virus. One scientist at the CDC in Atlanta noticed that one of the flasks that contained a mixture of Vero cells and throat tissue from a patient had turned from cloudy to clear. The clear areas meant that something was killing the Vero cells.

The flask material was processed so that it could be viewed under a special electron microscope, which magnified it over eighty thousand times. Many researchers believed that the microscopic view would show a pathogen from the family of viruses that cause various strains of flu. What they saw, however, was something they never expected: a coronavirus.

Coronaviruses are easily identifiable by their round shape crowned with what look like spikes under an electron microscope. (The viruses get their name from the Latin word *corona*, meaning "crown.") One reporter who viewed the viruses in a Hong Kong lab notes that "magnified 100,000 times, the organisms are fuzzy little balls that fill the screen and look like the burrs that stick to your pants during a hike through the woods. . . . You can just make out tiny hooks poking out of the spherical bodies."[29]

But while coronaviruses can make animals very sick and are often seen in livestock infections, in humans they had never been known to cause anything more serious than a cold. Never had scientists seen anything in the coronavirus family that could cause pneumonia or anything as deadly as this new disease.

## Trying Out a New Tool

The next step was to find out more about this particular coronavirus. To do that, WHO researchers sent samples of the virus to a laboratory at the University of California in San Francisco. Doctors there have a new tool called a DNA microarray, with which they can pinpoint a virus by examining a fragment of its genetic makeup.

The DNA microarray contains a slide spotted with fragments from over one thousand viruses known to science. If the WHO sample has any fragments that match up with the samples on the slide, spots will light up on a special scanning device. Then the army of spots is displayed on a computer monitor, and when a technician slides a cursor over any lit up spot, the name of the virus will pop up.

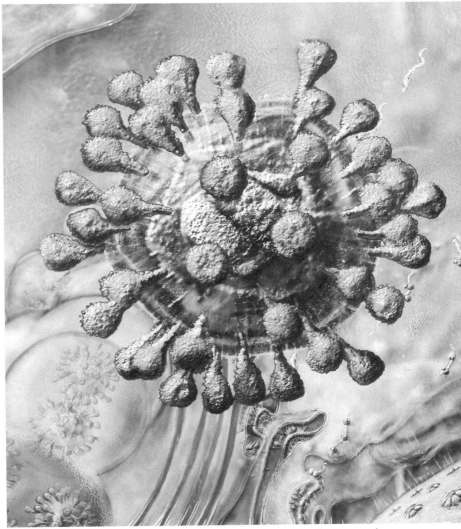

*The SARS virus is pictured inside a human cell. Scientists used a new tool called a DNA microarray to study the coronavirus that causes SARS.*

In this case, researchers were excited to see several spots light up on the microarray. The good news was that there were genetic similarities to three known coronaviruses that infect animals. The bad news was that the mystery virus was not identical to any of them. It was a new virus, never seen or studied.

## "Suddenly They're Rock Stars"

The scientific community realized that the dangerous unknown coronavirus was a problem. While there are many researchers who study viruses, there were not many who specialized in coronaviruses. One doctor says that because coronaviruses had never been a serious threat to people and were difficult to grow or study in a laboratory, the topic had become "a sleepy little corner of virology."[30] Far more researchers were interested in studying viruses that cause Ebola, West Nile disease, or AIDS—all of which are known killers. With the discovery of this particular virus, however, coronaviruses became a hot topic, and anyone

*A man suffers from Ebola in a hospital. Before discovering SARS, researchers neglected coronaviruses, focusing instead on the viruses responsible for such epidemics as Ebola and AIDS.*

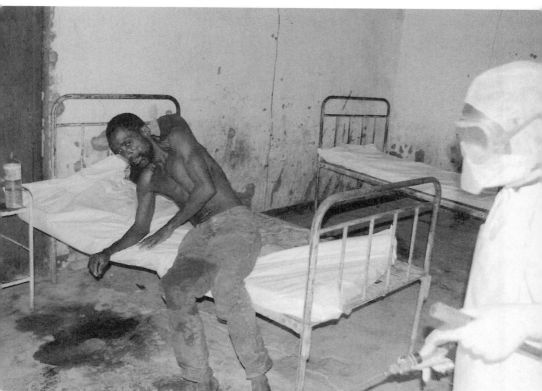

who specialized in them was in great demand. "Suddenly," laughs one virologist, "they're rock stars."[31]

After adding such specialists to the WHO team, researchers concentrated their efforts on the puzzling new coronavirus. Like others in its family, the SARS virus has spikes coated with proteins, which are designed to latch onto the cell of an organism—in this case, most likely an animal victim. The surfaces of an animal's cells have receptors, which are designed to link up with important body chemicals, such as insulin. A virus whose spikes match up with a cell's receptors can then latch onto the cell and infect the animal.

Once a cell is invaded by a coronavirus, the virus takes over the reproductive system of the cell and uses it to replicate itself—up to one thousand times per cell. This process eventually kills the cells, and the animal becomes sick. The key, says coronavirus expert Kathryn Holmes, is to find out how the SARS virus—whose genetic material most resembles an animal, not a human, virus—began infecting people in the first place. "We know the people getting SARS now are catching it from people, not from being exposed to unusual animals," said Holmes. "But where did it come from?"[32]

## Frustrating Mutations

Holmes and other experts believe it is likely that an animal virus mutated, and its protein spikes changed in such a way that they could latch onto human cells. Perhaps the barbs on the spikes altered in mutation, enabling them to be more of a threat to a human host. Researchers working on mapping the virus's genetic makeup support that theory, for in twelve different laboratories, twelve genetic profiles have been noted.

Researchers believe that the variety of genetic profiles is due to the primitive nature of coronaviruses. All known coronaviruses are composed of single strands of genetic material which has no built-in system to spot errors as it reproduces, as other viruses do. That means that every time the virus replicates itself, it changes in a very slight way. Notes one virologist, "Coronaviruses mutate for a living."[33]

This constant mutation is frustrating to scientists who are searching for a reliable tool for doctors to diagnose patients. In some diseases, doctors can perform blood tests to look for antibodies—the body's response to a particular germ that contains the genetic code of the virus. With an ever changing code, however, the coronavirus makes diagnosis tricky, for the antibodies in one patient may look different from those of another patient. "You look for symptoms like a cough, fatigue, a low-grade fever," says one doctor. "But that pretty much sums up a case of the flu, doesn't it? It's no wonder that so many SARS patients have been hospitalized in [regular hospital] wards, when they should have been isolated."[34]

## Returning to Guangdong

To find answers to the virus's beginnings, some researchers went to Guangdong Province, where the first cases of SARS occurred. Scientists noted that the first victims of the disease were people who worked in the many live animal markets throughout the province. A visit to a market just an hour south of the province's capital showed reporter Elizabeth Rosenthal a place that seemed rife with germs:

> In hundreds of cramped stalls that stink of blood and guts, wholesale food vendors tend to veritable zoos that will grace Guangdong Province's tables: snakes, chickens, cats, turtles, badgers, frogs. And, in summertime, sometimes rats, too. They are all stacked in cages one on top of another—which in turn serve as seats, card tables for the poor migrants who work there.[35]

Scientists found it easy to imagine how a virus could move from such animals to people in the crowded and filthy conditions of the market stalls, where sick and dying animals were cramped together in filthy cages in close proximity to stall workers. To test that theory, researchers collected specimens from eight different wild animals sold at the market and found varied strains of the coronavirus in all eight animals, including civet cats and rats being butchered in the stalls.

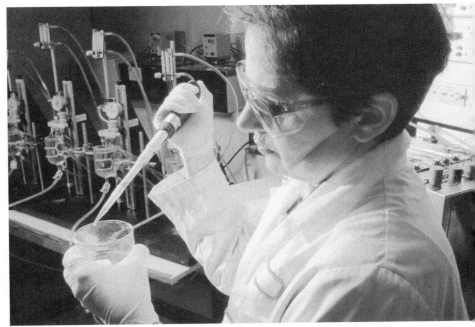

A scientist studies the SARS virus for clues about how it spreads from person to person. Scientists discovered that close contact is not necessary for transmission of the pathogen.

## From Person to Person

As some researchers concentrated on the beginnings of the virus and its probable jump from animals to people, others tried to understand how it spread from person to person. At first doctors believed that for someone with SARS to infect another person required fairly close proximity, with the infected person sneezing or coughing and those droplets coming into contact with an uninfected person.

However, as doctors began seeing more patients with SARS, they noticed that in all cases, the disease affects the lower part of a patient's lungs. That means that close contact is not necessary. Viruses that arise from the lower lungs tend to come out in a fine aerosol, rather than heavy droplets from sneezes and bronchial coughs. The aerosol is so light that it can linger for a much longer time in the air.

In addition, scientists found that the SARS virus can live outside the body for up to twenty-four hours, which means that it might be possible for an infected person who touches a doorknob or elevator button, for example, to leave an active virus for someone who touches those same objects hours later. That may explain, say scientists, how so many people were infected by one person at the Hong Kong hotel in March 2003.

*Because SARS is so contagious and because the virus can live outside the body for many hours, doctors must wear protective suits when treating infected patients.*

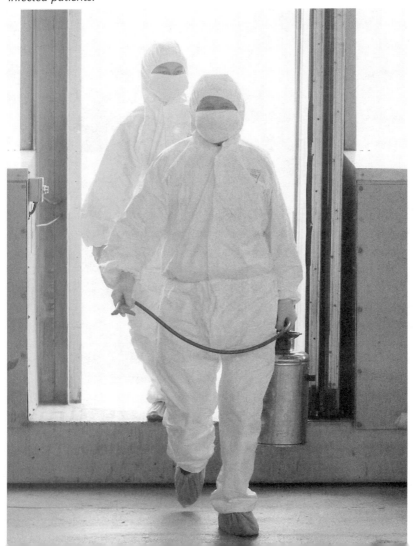

## A Puzzle

But even that theory could not account for the situation at the Amoy Gardens, a thirty-three-floor housing project in Hong Kong. In March 2003 clusters of people who had never met one another became infected. By the end of that month, three hundred people had become infected with SARS, and researchers scrambled to find an explanation for the rapid transmission of the disease. Said one WHO researcher in mid-March, "There is something going on—a form of transmission we don't understand."[36]

Some doctors in Hong Kong were frustrated by their inability to pinpoint the method of infection. They worried that the disease might even be spread through heating and cooling vents from one apartment to another. If that disturbing theory were true, it would be almost impossible to protect oneself from SARS if anyone in the building had it.

A more plausible theory was put forward in April. Researchers learned that a kidney patient left a Hong Kong hospital and visited his brother at the Amoy Gardens. Without realizing it, the kidney patient had become infected with SARS at the hospital, where many early SARS patients were treated. While at his brother's apartment, the infected man suffered from bouts of diarrhea, and used the toilet frequently. Researchers believe that it is possible that the SARS virus was spread throughout the Amoy Gardens by the man's feces.

Once flushed in the toilet, the virus-infected waste could have contaminated the sewage system through faulty plumbing. Rats, roaches, or other vermin could have come into contact with the virus in the leaky sewer pipe and carried it throughout the building, where hundreds of people unknowingly became infected. The theory is plausible, but residents of the Amoy Gardens remained nervous. "We don't really think [the doctors] know themselves what the method of transmission is," says one woman. "How do they know? It's just a theory, and no one is sure, and that is what makes me frightened."[37]

## Superspreaders?

Another puzzling aspect of the SARS epidemic are those people known as "superspreaders"—those who seem to be able to infect large numbers of people. From the beginning, scientists have been baffled at how one infected person can infect ninety people, while another can be ill without spreading the virus at all. Some researchers believe that people are superspreaders because of the way they cough—perhaps forcing more of the contaminated phlegm or spray from their lungs than do most patients. Others believe that some people have far more of the virus in their systems for some reason, and that makes them more likely to contaminate others.

On the other hand, researchers believe that some people who have had SARS have been able to fight off the virus without becoming ill. "I'm quite convinced that some people might have contracted the infection but not the disease," says one Hong Kong researcher. "Some may develop mild symptoms, like a little bit of cough and no fever; some may just feel a little tired for a day or two."[38]

This phenomenon is a mystery, just as the existence of superspreaders. Having people with the virus who do not become ill, however, is far more beneficial to the public. Scientists know that mild cases of SARS, where people do not exhibit any serious symptoms, are a good thing, because they act as natural vaccines. People lucky enough to get only a mild infection will have immunity from the virus in the future.

## No Cure in Sight

But for the majority of people, a case of SARS is a very serious threat—and one for which scientists have yet to find an effective cure. Treatment or prevention of the disease is an ongoing challenge, but doctors admit that there is much to be learned about the virus before cures are found. Until then, researchers hope that an existing drug for a different virus might give some relief.

In Hong Kong, for example, doctors have been giving some patients a combination of steroids and an antiviral drug called Ribavirin. Though they say it has had promising results in some cases, other researchers are doubtful because the drugs do not have an effect on the SARS virus in their labs. In other labs, re-

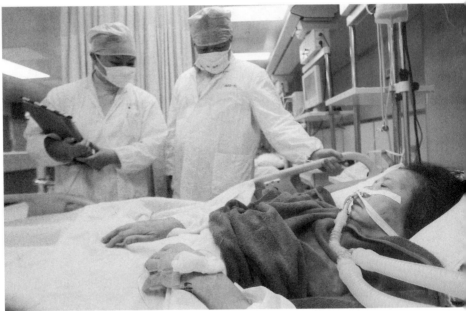

*Doctors treat a SARS patient in a Chinese hospital. Researchers continue to investigate new and effective ways to treat patients infected with the SARS virus.*

searchers are testing other drugs, such as those for hepatitis, AIDS, asthma, and some cancers. They hope that the same enthusiasm and spirit of cooperation the international science community showed in identifying the virus will cure the disease as well.

# Chapter 3

# Life with SARS

**S**ARS HAS HAD a dramatic effect on the way people go about their daily lives in places that have had outbreaks of the disease. Some of these changes have been merely inconvenient, while others serve as frightening reminders of how quickly a disease can turn life upside down—not only for those who are infected, but for healthy people, too.

## Clean Tires and Disinfectant

Once the Chinese government realized that it was necessary to openly confront the SARS epidemic, life changed quickly for the Chinese people. Interestingly, China's authoritarian system, which has been widely criticized as repressive, proved to be very useful in fighting the epidemic. "In a country where the government rules by fist," notes observer Kathy Chen, "its orders to fight [SARS] have been carried out in spades."[39]

For example, the state-run media were required to run public service programs several times each day, informing people how to minimize their risk of infection. Banners were put up in every city and village reminding people to wash their hands and wear face masks, and volunteers were rounded up to staff checkpoints for taking people's temperatures. Chinese officials even decreed that people must disinfect their bicycle and automobile tires each day to kill any germs that might have come home with them.

One man from a town in central China learned how strongly the government felt about containing SARS. Yang Jie, a twenty-two-year-old who worked for a home-improvement company in Beijing, decided to return home for a visit during the height of the epidemic. However, before being allowed on the train Yang had to undergo a thorough physical to make sure that he was not infected with SARS. During the fourteen-hour train trip, railroad workers came through his car several times to spray disinfectant. And when he arrived in his home town, Yang and several other passengers who had boarded the train in Beijing were put into quarantine for a week before being allowed to return to their families.

## "Are You Feeling Well Today?"

Travel restrictions were not limited to China, however. At the Singapore airport, all travelers getting off planes—regardless of their point of origin—were greeted by nurses wearing face masks, goggles, and protective yellow gowns cheerfully saying, "Welcome to Singapore! Are you feeling well today?"[40] The nurses then guided the passengers through high-tech scanners

*In an effort to prevent the spread of SARS, the Chinese government ordered citizens to take many precautions, including disinfecting their bicycles daily.*

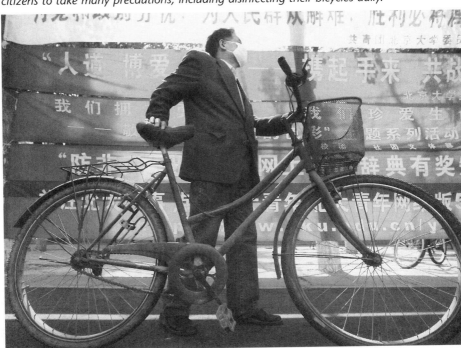

that would beep if a person had a fever of more than one hundred degrees. Anyone setting off the beeper was quickly escorted by masked soldiers to a video-camera–enforced quarantine area.

Singapore was serious about preventing travelers who might have SARS from coming into contact with its citizens. Anyone who balked at being quarantined was fitted with an electronic wristband, and anyone who persisted in trying to escape during the ten-day quarantine period was jailed for six months and fined five thousand dollars. "We do what we have to," explained Singapore's minister of health. "I don't think we've seen anything like this before, and it is a global problem. For now, this is a battle that is being fought with the thermometer and quarantine."[41]

In many countries around the world, governments enacted strong restrictions on visitors from a SARS-affected nation. Saudi Arabia simply refused to allow Asians or Canadians to enter the country. Thailand allowed travelers from China, Singapore, and Vietnam to visit, but required that they wear face masks for the duration of their stay.

After Canada experienced an outbreak of SARS, its health ministry requested a ten-day voluntary quarantine from any traveler from a SARS-affected nation. Those travelers were not required to go to a particular facility, as they were in Singapore, but were asked to stay at home, take their temperature every few hours, and to stay in a separate room from anyone else for ten days. By mid-April, there were believed to be at least seven thousand people in Canada under voluntary quarantine.

## Life in Quarantine

Some of those in quarantine were relatives and friends of people who had developed SARS. Many spent the required two-week period (the longest time known between being exposed to the disease and showing symptoms of it) at their homes. Besides being told to take their temperatures often and to stay away from their families, they had to resist the temptation of dashing out to do an errand or see a friend.

Thousands of others were put on what was called "working quarantine." Most of these were health care workers who had

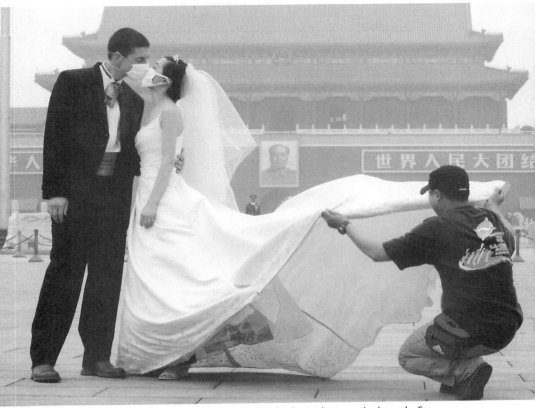

*A New York man kisses his Chinese bride through a surgical mask. Some visitors to China and to other countries impacted by SARS were forced to spend up to two weeks in quarantine.*

been exposed to SARS at North York General or Scarborough Grace Hospitals—the two facilities that treated the SARS patients during the epidemic and which later transferred all patients except those with SARS to other hospitals in the city. Those workers at Scarborough or North York who had been exposed were allowed to work their regular shift—wearing masks and protective gear—but afterward had to return home.

Peggy Dawson, a twenty-nine-year-old nurse who works at Scarborough Grace Hospital, was put on working quarantine, though she says that to the best of her knowledge, she was not exposed to anyone with SARS for the period in question. "However, there were other members of the staff," she said, "who could have been exposed, from people who clean the floors to physiotherapists and respiratory therapists. We all share the same cafeteria, come in through the same entrance. It's a contact of a contact, and that's why we are all under quarantine, the entire hospital."[42] Dawson says that every day she worried that she would develop symptoms. "Every time I put the thermometer in my mouth," she admitted, "I'm praying that there isn't a change." She has remained healthy, but says that even though she is out of quarantine she still worries that an epidemic—SARS or something else—will happen again. "It has really changed the face of nursing," says Dawson, "and changed the face of health care forever."[43]

## "It Feels like Being in Prison"

Quarantine was often far different for people in Asia. Shortly after it was discovered that more than 250 residents of the large Hong Kong housing complex, the Amoy Gardens, had become infected with SARS, health officials descended on Block E of the complex and bused the 240 remaining residents to quarantine facilities.

Many of the evacuees were angry, however, for they say that their temporary lodging seemed far more conducive to the spread of disease than their housing complex. The facilities to which they were taken were rundown resort settlements, which were cramped and filthy. One woman says that she spent the first morning in quarantine disinfecting her cabin's toilet with bleach—only to be told that several families would be sharing bathrooms during the quarantine. Said the woman, "It feels like being in prison."[44]

In the eastern mainland province of Zhejiang, SARS patients were quarantined in a government office building. Not only were those quarantined angry at the lack of facilities—no beds, for example—but nonquarantined residents staged violent protests at the use of those buildings. Breaking windows and smashing furniture, townspeople were furious that such buildings were used, calling the quarantine a danger to everyone. They worried that after the quarantine ended, germs would remain in the buildings, endangering citizens. Insisted one protester, "They shouldn't have hospitalized patients in the government building, which has no medical facilities and professional staff."[45]

## Reminders Everywhere

Though SARS patients and others quarantined were most affected, daily life—even for healthy people—changed drastically during the SARS crisis in China and other Asian countries. For children in Singapore and China, it meant that school was canceled until the threat of infection had passed. For parents of very young children, it meant babysitting services, daycares, and preschools were closed, too. That presented a problem for people who had no older children or other family members to watch their young children while they went to work. In Singapore alone, more than six hundred thousand young children were affected by the closing of child care services.

There were daily bulletins on radio and television that gave the totals of new infections and numbers of deaths for the day. In these bulletins parents were strongly urged not to take their children to public places such as the zoo, playgrounds, or shopping malls. One woman says that it was especially hard on children who were celebrating birthdays during this time. Parties had to be canceled. It was probably for the best, she says, since no one felt like celebrating.

Lest anyone forget—even for a moment—that there was a dangerous disease in the area, there were constant reminders everywhere one looked. "Security officers stationed at the driveway of our apartment building were stopping everyone," one woman says, "even cabdrivers, to take their temperatures."[46]

In Singapore, every business person was stopped before entering a downtown building and, before using the elevator, had to fill out a health evaluation form. People were afraid of buses and trains because of the threat of touching a contaminated door or seat. Instead of relying on public transportation as is usual in most Asian cities, people opted to ride their bicycles—a decision that created massive traffic jams.

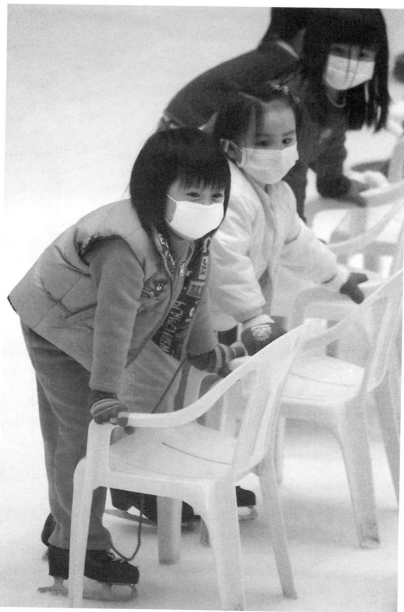

*Children in Hong Kong wear masks to protect against SARS. These masks were in high demand in China as people took precautions to avoid contracting the disease.*

## Bambi and Teddy Bear Masks

More than anything else, however, it was the presence of face masks that served as a constant reminder of the threat of SARS. People rushed to medical supply stores to buy them, hoping to keep airborne germs away from their noses and mouths. In Hong Kong, stores were selling more than one thousand masks each day—some people were buying hundreds at a time. When only a few were left on store shelves, shouting matches often broke out among customers.

On street corners, vendors tried to capitalize on the frenzy. On a Singapore street, a vendor sold turquoise masks with pictures of Bambi or a teddy bear on them. They appealed to parents whose small children did not like wearing face masks. "My kids don't want to wear them," said one mother as she bought two of the Bambi masks. "With cartoons on them, they might change their minds."[47]

Masks seemed to be everywhere SARS was. They were worn by bank tellers, flight attendants, and waiters. Even on television, talk show hosts (and their guests) wore masks, too. But the mask-wearing has brought up some new issues of etiquette that have never been considered before. For example, business people debate whether masks make their clients more or less afraid. Should one remove one's mask when meeting someone for the first time? And since touching and handshakes are frowned upon in the age of SARS, how best to greet a valued customer or client?

Cab drivers in Hong Kong and Singapore found that because they wore masks, they were losing business. As a result, many opted not to wear them and left their windows open instead. Too, there was the issue of comfort; the most effective masks are form-fitting, and they can cause discomfort when worn for hours at a time. They are also hard to breathe through when exercising or doing strenuous work. One American visitor to China felt that the mask was more trouble than it was worth. "I wear my masks most places," he said, "but it's uncomfortable because it's humid here, and in a restaurant when you're trying to eat, it's just impractical."[48]

## Fear Among Health Workers

While the constant worry about SARS was hard on almost everyone, it was especially troubling for health care workers. They were the ones most at risk, and in the early weeks of the disease, it was doctors and nurses in mainland China, Hong Kong, Vietnam, and Toronto who were infected more than any other group.

Because of the shortage of healthy emergency workers in Toronto, Canadian physicians contacted doctors they knew in the United States and asked for help. As a result, about three hundred American doctors agreed to come to Toronto. The Canadian government issued temporary medical licenses to the Americans (physicians are normally allowed to practice medicine only in the country from which they received their medical license.)

One of the American doctors who traveled to Canada says that the atmophere in the Toronto hospital where she worked was both angry and frightened. So little was known about SARS—especially how it was transmitted—that health workers felt vulnerable even with protective gear. The healthy members of the staff were burned-out because they had to work more shifts to cover for their colleauges who had caught SARS or who were in quarantine. Many were working double or even triple shifts. "They're not getting enough sleep, they struggle with putting on their protective gear," said the chief of infectious diseases at the University of Toronto, "and they are worried about getting infected themselves."[49]

## "Mommy, Are You Wearing Your Mask?"

Trish Perl, one of the American doctors who came to help in Toronto, noticed right away that there was a strange atmosphere at the hospital, with everyone wearing layers of protective gear—even in the staff lounges. Some moved to the other end of a meeting room when a doctor who had cared for a SARS patient walked in. "It was eerie—like you were on Mars or on a new planet," she says. "You sit in meetings, everyone around the table is wearing an N-95 [high-quality face] mask."[50]

Perl was struck, too, by the number of doctors and clinical workers who are so afraid of SARS that they cannot—or will

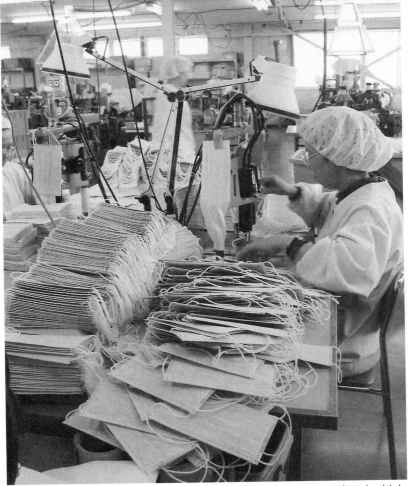

*Throughout the first half of 2003, medical supply companies produced a high volume of surgical masks to meet soaring worldwide demand.*

not—deal directly with patients with symptoms that might be SARS. For example, she noted that some would not deal with anyone with a fever of more than one hundred degrees, or who suffered from a dry cough. One radiologist stayed in his office with his door closed and refused to have any contact with X-ray technicians. The only X-rays he would read were those slipped under his door.

Perl admits that she was fearful before she traveled to Canada, since she was unsure of how bad the situation was. Like other physicians, she was concerned about the many health care workers who had become infected—even though they had taken precautions. "As I was hugging my little girl on leaving, I thought,

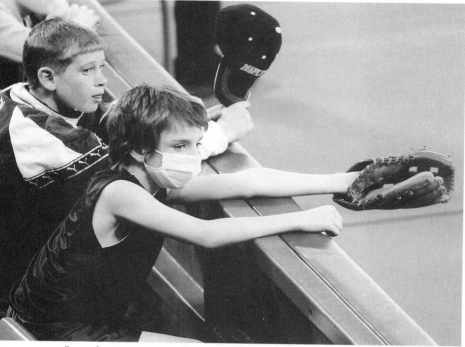

*Fear of contracting SARS reached as far as Toronto, Canada, after several cases of the disease were reported there. Here, a boy wears a surgical mask to a Bluejays game.*

'What am I doing?'" Perl remembers. "'Is this a smart thing to do?' I was very scared at first; I didn't know what I was getting into." And when she talked to her children on the telephone, she was not surprised at what they wanted to know. "They would say, 'Mommy, are you wearing your mask?'"[51]

## Hungry Ghosts

SARS has not only changed the routine for doctors and hospitals, but for the families of the victims of SARS. For instance, the disease has forced a change in the cultural rituals associated with death. In China, for example, people are expected to remain with a dying family member. A family vigil, known as *you zi song zong*, is considered extremely important to ensure that after death, the spirit is happy. However, when SARS spread to Hong Kong, doctors began to realize how vulnerable family members and other visitors were as they sat with an infected patient. By the end of March 2003 most hospitals in Hong Kong prohibited visits by family members. This meant no vigils, and families were upset.

Vigils are important for more than support for a dying loved one. Many Asian people believe that it is important to note the expression of a person's face at the moment of death. Families believe that a person who dies with open mouth or open eyes dies trying to communicate something important. To have a loved one die in such distress can produce guilt within a family that can last for many years. The spirits of those who have died with such unfinished business are called "hungry ghosts," and are greatly feared. "People who have died an early death—from a disease or other natural causes—are considered dangerous," explains anthropologist Joseph Bosco. "They've got every right to be angry at the world, because they were cheated out of their

*Because scientists were initially uncertain how SARS spreads, finding funeral homes to perform services for people who died from the disease was difficult.*

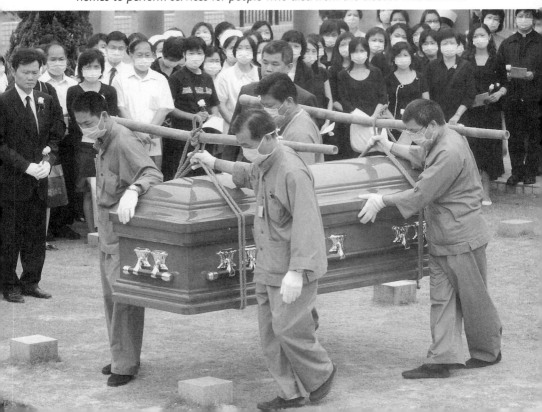

lives."[52] And because of the hospitals' need to keep family members separated from the dying SARS patients, people do not know the emotional state in which their loved ones died.

## Cold and Empty

Because people were unsure of how SARS was spread, families had a great deal of difficulty finding funeral parlors that would accept a SARS victim's body—and even those refused to hold traditional funeral services. Throughout Asia, funerals are almost always held with the body displayed, but the threat of SARS changed that. Funeral directors, worried about spreading the disease from the dead body to funeral guests, insisted on using a framed photograph of the deceased, instead.

Another funeral custom that has been suspended because of SARS is the ceremonial "water buying," in which a family member—usually the oldest son or male relative—purchases water with which to wash the dead person's face. This symbolic ritual is extremely important to many Asian people—so much so, says one funeral director in Hong Kong, that "among the older generation in Hong Kong, the greatest insult would be to say, 'When you die, I hope you have no sons to buy you water.'"[53]

Not surprisingly, the funerals for SARS victims tend to be sparsely attended, which is disappointing to grieving families that need the support of others. One woman says she felt terrible when only a handful of her husband's friends showed up for his funeral. "I felt the atmosphere was cold and empty," she says. "I was broken down spiritually and psychologically."[54]

## The Psychological Toll

As months went by in SARS-affected countries, many learned that there were often psychological effects on residents. In Hong Kong, for example, many people complained of feeling mentally fatigued each day. There was no comfort of routine. There were no concerts to attend, no social get-togethers with neighbors.

Many people found that the sources from which they had always drawn strength were missing. For some it was religion, and there were noticeable changes in churches in Asia and Canada. In

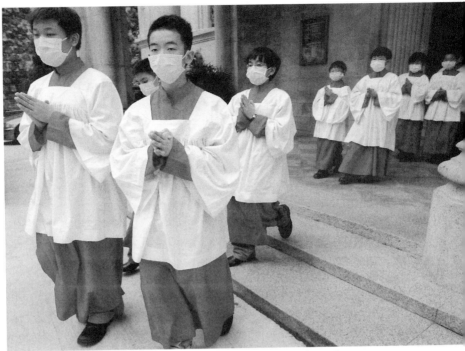

*Altar boys attend Catholic mass in Hong Kong. Churches throughout areas impacted by SARS welcomed parishioners struggling with the emotional effects of the epidemic.*

Singapore, for example, the Catholic Church suspended confessions in private confessional booths—instead offering general forgiveness to their parishioners. Toronto churchgoers were asked not to dip their hands in holy water or to share wine at communion.

Others in SARS-affected regions missed the support they normally received from their families. Since many foreign business people in Asia had moved their families to other continents in an attempt to avoid SARS, they weathered the ordeal without the comfort of their spouse and children. Karl Taro Greenfield, a *Time* magazine reporter living in Hong Kong, says the experience was not just a medical threat but one that affected people's spirits. "The quesions raised alter the rhythm of life itself," he noted. "Do you dare dine communally, as is the custom here in Hong

Kong? Is it safe to work out at the gym? If you do work out, is it advisable to take a shower in the clubhouse afterward? Do you kiss your children?"[55]

One man said that people put a huge importance on daily radio and television bulletins about SARS, hoping to hear promising news about the disease. "Every evening, the Department of Health releases the numbers of new infections and fatalities," he said. "If the numbers are lower than yesterday, we cling to the hope the worst is over. If there are more new cases and deaths, we shudder."[56]

## Psychiatric Study

For people who have survived SARS, the psychological toll has been documented. In a study of 150 SARS patients in Hong Kong, it has been found that 45 suffered from psychiatric problems when they were discharged from the hospital. The problems have ranged from anxiety and mild depression to episodes of posttraumatic stress and severe panic attacks. Some doctors suggest that the psychiatric problems may stem from a reaction to the steroids and other drugs given in the hospital, but no one is certain.

*The fear of SARS became an overriding factor in the lives of many Chinese, who paid anxious attention to news reports, hoping for promising news about the disease.*

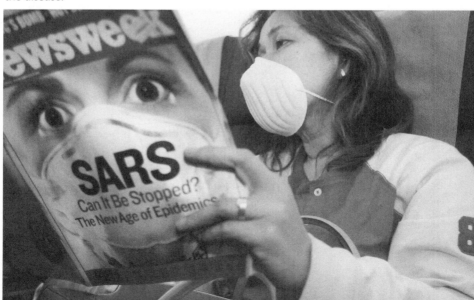

Health care workers who survived SARS, experts say, tend to be more fearful than before they were infected, and that as a result, they have not returned to their jobs as quickly as predicted. "We're finding that [because of the psychological factors] it takes quite a long time for some people to get back," says one Toronto doctor, "even if they haven't been that badly infected."[57]

One key factor that experts believe is contributing to the psychological problems of survivors is the stigma that is attached to them by society. Many patients found that employers were not willing to have them return to work because they believed the survivors remained a high risk for infecting others in the workplace. One Hong Kong woman was fired after refusing to sign a vow to break up with her boyfriend—a health care emergency worker.

Not only recovered patients, but also many doctors, nurses, friends, and relatives of patients have been ostracized, too. One Hong Kong woman who lives at the Amoy Gardens residence was shunned not only by friends but by her own family—even though her area of the housing complex was not affected by SARS or the quarantine. The fear of SARS was so strong that neither her mother nor her eight brothers and sisters would see her, and she was treated as an outcast at work.

Her experience is not uncommon; in fact, Hong Kong's minister of health finally reacted to the lack of empathy by the public toward people remotely affected by SARS, urging people to be less fearful and more compassionate. Even so, by June 2003, the Hong Kong Equal Opportunities Commission had received thirty-eight complaints of SARS-related discrimination, and officials believed there would be more filed within the month. Because so little was understood about the disease, those who had been infected and had survived often remained on society's periphery.

# Chapter 4

# SARS, Politics, and the Economy

WHILE PEOPLE AROUND the world were trying to deal with the treatment and containment of the disease, civic and national leaders were dealing with other aspects of SARS. Of particular concern was the way a new contagious disease affected the economy and politics of places that had suffered large outbreaks of SARS.

## Nothing New

China was not honest about the SARS outbreak in providing information about the mysterious disease to the international medical community. In addition, the government was equally dishonest to its own citizens about SARS. China's history contains stories of several empires that were toppled because of uprisings by the masses. Lest they suffer the same fate, modern Chinese leaders have tried to keep frightening events such as the SARS epidemic a secret. By the government's decision not to be truthful, say experts, Chinese leaders were continuing a troubling tradition of covering up the nation's medical problems.

For example, in the late 1990s there was a large outbreak of HIV, the virus that causes AIDS, in the rural areas of central China. The disease spread among people who had sold their blood to traffickers, using needles and other equipment tainted with the virus. As a result, tens of thousands of people became infected with HIV, though the government insisted that only a handful of people in a remote village were affected by the traffickers' carelessness.

Another example of governmental secrecy occurred in early 2003, when more than three thousand schoolchildren in a northeastern province became ill—and three died—after drinking spoiled soy milk. Again, though thousands of parents were seeking medical help for their children, the government denied that any such thing had happened. As a result of instances such as these, the government suffered a lack of credibility when people eventually learned that their leaders had not been honest with them.

## Angry Doctors

Similarly, many people feel that China's government may suffer because of its lack of openness with its citizens about the SARS virus. Once word of the disease began to leak out, many Chinese

*Healthcare workers like this man were angry with the Chinese government for its initial refusal to provide information about the extent of the SARS epidemic.*

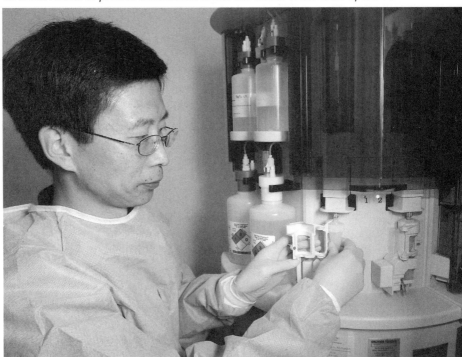

citizens felt that they had been duped. Many of the angriest people were health care workers.

To make the numbers of infected people seem low, government health officials decreed in March 2003 that doctors could no longer diagnose SARS; instead, for a diagnosis to be official, it must be made by a medical researcher. But because researchers were unable to see even one-fourth of the patients suspected of having the disease, many patients whom doctors suspected of having SARS went undiagnosed.

One doctor in Shanghai recalls a patient he saw whose symptoms almost certainly indicated SARS. He says that he wanted to isolate the patient and begin treating his fever and cough, but before he could begin, he was stunned to find that his patient had been transferred without his knowledge. "I never found out whether he had the disease or not," says the doctor. "We doctors are all left with a lot of questions. I think it's shameful to not let us know what's going on."[58]

## Misinformation

But it is not just medical workers who are angry at the government's secrecy. It is almost certain that thousands of Chinese people became ill, some fatally, because they were not told about the seriousness of the disease. One man says that the government had assured everyone that the risk of SARS was long over, even when health officials knew that the disease was spreading out of control. As a result of the misinformation, the man says, his wife was ill and highly contagious for days with SARS—and the family was certain it must be something else.

Chinese journalists, who are largely under the control of the Communist Party, admit that they were used by the government to convince the public that SARS was not a problem. In Shanghai, for example, journalists were told that the number of people in the city with SARS was highly classified and were warned that they would be fired or jailed if they attempted to interview SARS patients or their families.

At the same time, however, health officials were worried that unless they educated the public about the symptoms of SARS, they would be unable to contain the outbreak in Shanghai, whose population is 16 million. One journalist recalls that his orders from government officials were highly contradictory. "Readers are going to be very confused," he tried to explain to the province's health minister. "On the one hand, we tell them there are almost no cases in Shanghai. On the other, we tell them that they must be very vigilant in avoiding the disease. But if Shanghai has barely any cases, why does the public have to be worried about SARS?"[59]

## "The Government Doesn't Care"

Of course, in busy cities like Shanghai and Beijing the ballooning rate of infection from SARS was hard to keep secret. As more and more people learned of friends and coworkers who had become infected, it became clear to the public that they had been lied to. Many were furious with their government. "It's really bad," says a relative of a SARS victim, "that the government doesn't care about ordinary people's lives."[60]

As the disease moved into the more remote parts of China, the response was no less angry. The tiny remote villages have limited hospital facilities—a shortage which is troublesome under normal circumstances. They lack around-the-clock staff, X-ray machines, and even bed space for more than two or three patients at a time. When people infected with SARS began appearing at these rural hospitals, health workers were forced to turn many patients away. This experience showed residents the inadequacies of their health care system.

In one village, five or more SARS patients were crammed into a single ward room which had no door or even a curtain to stop the spread of germs. Since the hospital staff is minimal, family members were encouraged to stay with the patients. Because SARS was not supposed to be a problem, however, there was a shortage of face masks, and the families were constantly at risk of catching the disease. "We relatives have to stay in that room without any protective measures, all day and all night," complained one young man. "It's very dangerous, but we have no choice, if we want to take care of our family."[61]

## "Why Didn't the Government Say Anything?"

If this situation had occurred in the United States or any other democracy, it would hardly be surprising for people's anger to be directed at the government. However, China is a nation where power is monopolized by the Communist Party. Though it is very modern in its economic policies, China's political system has a long history of being resistant to change. The system is closed and secretive, and has a dismal record regarding human rights. Protesters have been shot for criticizing the government or its actions, and as a result, people tend to keep their anger or frustration to themselves.

*Two women try to keep SARS out by blocking the entrance to their village. Such remote rural areas lacked the facilities and resources to properly treat SARS patients.*

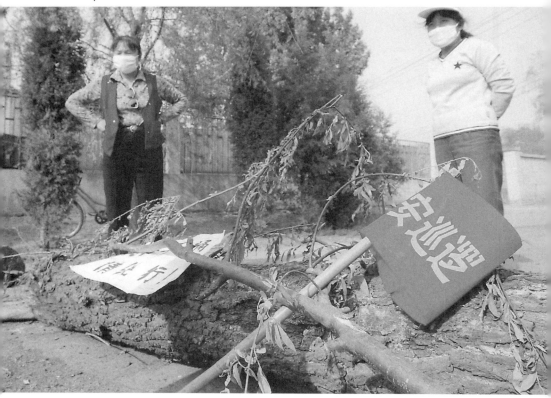

But people have been outspoken—many for the first time—about their government's mishandling of the SARS epidemic. One young woman who became infected after tending to her mother and father in the hospital when they had the disease was angry. "If we had known about this disease, we would have stayed away from the hospital," she says. "Why didn't the government say anything? I blame them for my parents' death."[62]

Many Chinese, fearing for the health of their families, felt that the government was less interested in preventing SARS than in keeping up the pretense that all was well in China's cities. In Beijing, for example, people were frantically trying to find transportation out of the city as shops and restaurants were closing because of the SARS threat. When officials urged people to stay home, they were ignored. "I'm very worried about getting on a train with so many people," said one young man in April 2003. "But I'll do anything to get out of Beijing. It's simply become too dangerous."[63]

At Beijing University, students openly rebelled against governmental orders to stay on campus during the height of the epidemic. University officials warned students that they would suffer consequences—including expulsion—if they left. Even so, many students packed their backpacks and left, hoping to avoid catching SARS. One student said that his classmates did not want to have their fate controlled by the government, explaining: "They said they'd have the control over their own legs."[64]

## "For the Sake of the People"

Much of the anger has been directed at China's new president, Hu Jintao. Hu, whose ideas are more liberal than his predecessors, had impressed many people in his first presidential speech, for he seemed more committed to honesty and openness than other leaders had been. He vowed to remember that the well-being of China's people was his most important responsibility: "Power must be used for the sake of the people," he urged. "Material benefits must be sought in the interests of the people."[65]

However, in the early days of the epidemic Hu allowed government health officials free rein in handling the crisis. They

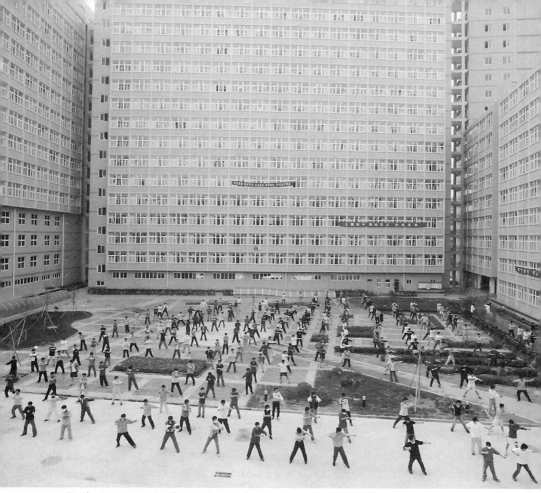

*Students quarantined at Beijing University do morning exercises. Many students defied government orders and left the campus to avoid contracting SARS.*

chose to deal with the disease in more traditional ways—in this case, being secretive about the severity of SARS. It was only when WHO and the international media became involved that Hu realized that he and his government were rapidly losing the trust of the people—in addition to that of the international community.

On April 20, 2003, Hu abruptly fired his health minister, replacing him with a no-nonsense former trade minister, Wu Yi. Wu's job was one-dimensional—to head the anti-SARS fight in China. It seemed clear that for the first time in memory, China's government was serious about openly confronting a crisis.

## The Black Box or the Sunshine

Hu's supporters were very pleased by his actions. They believed that his decision to be more open about SARS would benefit the nation. Perhaps, they said, this episode forced China to turn a corner, allowing much-needed reforms. "This is [Hu's] chance to grab the support of the people and stand up on his own," said one former party official. "China can keep living in a black box, or it can live in the sunshine. If he can't take advantage of the situation and move into the sun now, then when?"[66]

There is strong opposition to Hu's openness, however. Some Communist Party officials are critical of Hu's more liberal views. They predicted that his more open dealing with SARS would backfire, causing panic among the Chinese people. The former president of China, a conservative named Jiang Zemin, is one of the most adamant critics of Hu, and experts in Chinese politics predicted that if the SARS epidemic had not been controlled, Jiang might have regained power. If that had happened, say experts, it would have signaled a return to the more repressive regimes of past years.

No one doubts that the SARS issue was a political challenge for the Hu presidency. "For the Chinese government," noted one observer, "the SARS crisis presents the gravest threat since the student protests at Tiananmen Square [that resulted in more than 165 deaths of Chinese demanding democracy] fourteen years ago."[67]

## Economic Disaster

Politics is not the only thing that has been affected by SARS. In SARS-stricken countries, the epidemic has had a great economic impact—especially in China. Having recently won the rights to host the 2008 Olympics in Beijing, as well as the World Expo 2010 in Shanghai, Chinese economists were very pleased with the prospects for higher employment rates and rising stock prices. However, on April 2, 2003, when WHO declared Guangdong Province and Hong Kong danger zones, that optimism evaporated almost overnight.

The first setback was the sharp drop in the number of tourists. China depends on tourism, for it accounts for 9 percent of the economy. In both 2000 and 2001 the tourist industry accounted for $67 billion. After word of the SARS outbreak spread, however, tourists looked elsewhere for places to visit. In April 2003, alone, there were ten thousand cancellations for flights and hotel bookings because of people's fear of becoming infected with SARS. By July 2003 it was estimated that tourism would bring in 40 percent less money for the year.

There were cancellations of business-related events, too. Many foreign business representatives canceled meetings that had been scheduled to take place in China. A survey of business travel groups found that many of the airlines that have regular business flights to China had reported drops in sales. Explained one American financial representative in Shanghai, "Anything that requires face-to-face meetings is on hold."[68]

Trade shows, at which various companies show off new products for foreign buyers, were canceled. The few shows that went on as planned were poorly attended. The sales manager for one communications equipment company says that he always works long hours at the Taipei International Spring Show, at which he normally gets many orders. However, in the spring 2003 show he made so few sales he expects that his business will drop by at least 20 percent. "Most of my buyers didn't come this year,"[69] he says.

## Trickling Down

The loss of orders for factories, as well as the loss of revenue from tourism, had what economists call a "trickle-down effect" to other areas of the Chinese economy. In other words, it was not simply the factory owners or the hotel and restaurant owners who made less money. In fact, the brunt of the hardship fell not on the owners, but on the millions of people who work in those businesses.

In China and other Asian countries affected by SARS, the huge decrease in factory orders resulted in layoffs of millions of workers. Many of the factories affected were foreign-owned assembly plants that had moved their operations to Asia to save money, for factory workers in Asia are paid only a small fraction of what

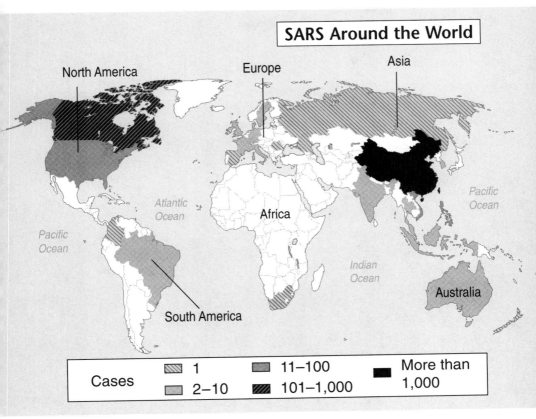

**SARS Around the World**

North America

Europe

Asia

Atlantic
Ocean

Africa

Pacific
Ocean

Pacific
Ocean

Indian
Ocean

Australia

South America

Cases

1    11–100    More than
2–10  101–1,000  1,000

such workers would earn in the United States or other nations. And several businesses that had been considering relocating to Asia were rethinking their plans, as owners wondered about the safety of a region suffering such a dangerous epidemic.

As restaurants and hotels stood empty, they, too, laid off large numbers of waiters, housekeepers, cooks, and cleaners. And without markets for their products, farmers and ranchers were affected, as the prices for produce and beef continued to drop. Experts say that the millions of new unemployed workers added a heavy strain to the already high jobless rate.

## Trouble for Hong Kong

Mainland China has been hard hit by the economic effects of the SARS epidemic, but Hong Kong has had even worse trouble.

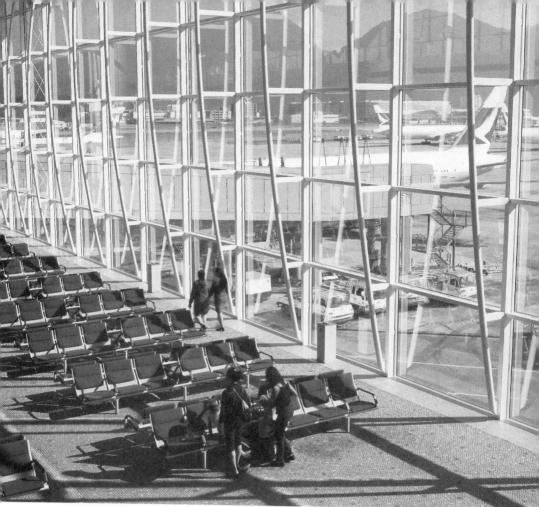

*As fear of SARS intensified, tourists canceled trips to Hong Kong, leaving the city's airport (pictured) empty and causing severe economic distress.*

Hong Kong, far and away the most modern part of China, had been experiencing economic difficulties even before the SARS crisis. It is a very expensive city; foreign firms with branches in Asia had found it so expensive for its employees to live there that many of the firms had relocated to the mainland. WHO's warning about visiting Hong Kong was even more damaging.

Within three weeks of the April 2 warning by WHO, Hong Kong's economic experts were fearing the worst. In 2002 more than a million Americans had visited the city, but it was clear that 2003 would be far different. Airlines that normally have several international flights each day to Hong Kong cut service drastically. The largest carrier to Hong Kong, Cathay Pacific, reduced its weekly flights by 45 percent almost immediately after news of the SARS outbreak became known. Hong Kong's airport, normally the fifth busiest in the world, was a virtual ghost town, writes one observer, "a series of vast, sparsely occupied and nearly silent halls, where travelers in surgical masks move quickly to and from gates."[70]

Business diminished in Hong Kong to a greater extent than on China's mainland. One local textile and furniture manufacturer says that 80 percent of foreign investors and buyers canceled buying trips—and that means a sharp loss of revenue for him, as well as a drastic loss of jobs for his workers. As with Mainland China, unemployed workers meant fewer dollars being spent by the citizens of Hong Kong. By May 2003 retail sales in Hong Kong had fallen 50 percent from the May 2002 totals.

## The Whole Region Contracts

The SARS epidemic has not only affected Chinese workers but also many foreigners who live and work in China. For example, more than 25 percent of American employees in Beijing sent their families out of the country because of the disease. One Australian bank with branch offices in Asia gave its employees in Hong Kong the option of returning to Australia—and were surprised when the majority said yes. A bank officer predicted that even when SARS is no longer a threat, many of those employees may decide to stay in Australia rather than risk working in Asia again. "You've got most of the [foreign] population [away from Asia] already, the families at least," he said, "and if this goes on, people will start to say, 'Why don't you relocate me [out of Asia where their families are]?'"[71]

More than thirty-four hundred miles away, Australian fishermen have been affected by the economic calamity in China, too. Those who fish along the Great Barrier Reef are feeling the loss of a great deal of their business due to the SARS outbreak. Their biggest customers are the restaurants in Hong Kong, and with the city's best restaurants closed because of SARS, there are no orders for their fish. As a result, many of Australia's fishing boats are idle, and their owners without jobs.

And though there have been relatively few SARS cases in the United States, Americans have been affected by the disease, too. By May 2003 the Federal Reserve announced that the economic problems throughout Asia were having effects in the United States. The stock market, which was already weakened by the uncertainty of the war effort in Iraq, showed that stock prices fell even further as banks and insurance companies that dealt with Asia lost business. One business owner notes that the decline in

*A woman passes a poster urging Shanghai residents to help check the spread of SARS by refraining from spitting. Spitting has been a socially acceptable practice in China for centuries.*

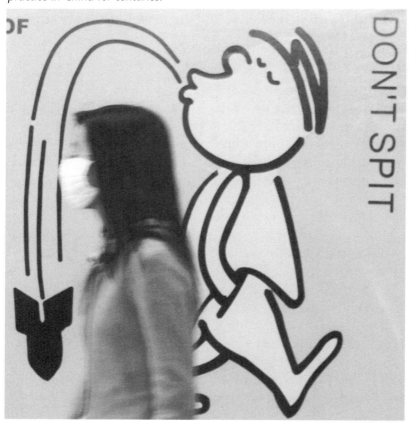

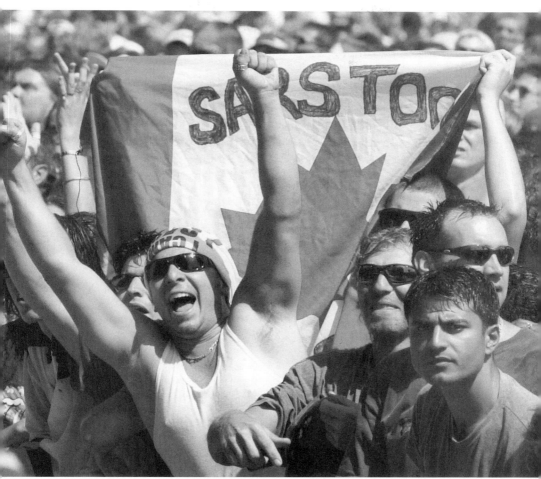

*A group of Canadians cheers at a 2003 benefit concert in Toronto aimed at raising money to help the local economy, devastated by SARS.*

airline travel alone made the business world skittish. "Just as business got used to the idea of the globe being a village," he says, "along comes a virus that affects something as fundamental to business as travel itself."[72]

## Canada Disagrees with WHO

While Asia was hit hardest by the political and economic fallout from SARS, Canada suffered, too. Because of the outbreak in

Toronto, which had infected more than 240 people, WHO added Canada to its list of global danger spots on April 23, 2003. That prompted a storm of outrage—not toward Canada's leaders but the World Health Organization itself.

The morning after the warning was issued, the United Nations received protests from Canada's prime minister as well as its health minister, saying that they did not agree with WHO labeling Toronto unsafe, nor did they accept the process that the organization followed. Toronto's mayor, Mel Lastman, appeared on television, both praising the health workers of the city and criticizing WHO for what he considered a lapse of judgment. "Let me be clear," he said in late April 2003. "It's safe to come to Toronto."[73]

Although the travel alert was lifted after one week, Canadian officials felt that the damage had already been done. Like China, Canada's economy depends on tourism, and economic analysts estimated that the SARS threat cost Canada a minimum of $30 million per day of the alert. A milder caution by WHO, listing Toronto as a SARS-impacted area, remained until July 2, 2003, and that definitely hurt not only Toronto's economy, but that of the entire nation.

Even in places such as Montreal and western Canada's Lake Louise and Banff National Park, where there were no cases of SARS, there were sharp declines in the number of visitors. One hotel official says that it is unfortunate that the public had the impression that Canada was dangerous because of SARS, when in reality, Toronto's health officials did a good job of containing the threat. "Perception versus reality was just so skewed," he says. "In terms of having a regular summer [of tourism], we're past that point."[74]

## An Impact on Baseball

Major league baseball in Toronto suffered, too. WHO's warning came just as the Toronto Blue Jays' season was getting underway, and league officials were hesitant to allow the season to go on as scheduled. Many teams who were supposed to travel to Toronto to play baseball were nervous when baseball league officials warned visiting players not to mingle with fans or sign auto-graphs.

Although baseball officials agreed that most likely the chance of a player catching SARS in Toronto was small, they maintained it was important for players to be careful. One player agreed, saying that as long as people were still contracting SARS, it made sense for players to be cautious. "I think right now we have to back off a little bit," he said, "and make sure everybody stays safe until they find out what's going on. I think [fans] should under-stand what's going on, because people are dying from this thing. It's not like people are just sick. People have died."[75]

# Chapter 5

# SARS and the Future

ON JULY 6, 2003, the World Health Organization announced that SARS had been contained, as no new cases of the disease had been reported anywhere in the world since June 15. Although the announcement was a relief to many people, medical experts tended to be less optimistic.

For instance, some felt that the disease could easily return. Because SARS is a coronavirus, it may be seasonal like other coronaviruses—such as those that cause the common cold. Michael Osterholm, director of the Center of Infectious Diseases at the University of Minnesota, felt a recurrence of SARS was not only possible, but likely. "I am convinced with the advent of an early winter in the Northern Hemisphere in just six short months," he told Congress, "we will see a resurgence of SARS that could far exceed our experience to date."[76]

Other infectious disease experts concurred, saying that it would only take one case of SARS to spark a new outbreak. And since it was impossible to know whether or not a person with SARS may have been misdiagnosed with some other ailment, an outbreak could come at any time. David Heymann of WHO agreed that it was crucial for doctors to be vigilant, saying, "It's very important countries continue their surveillance for at least the next twelve months."[77]

## "I'm a Bit Astounded"

Even if the SARS virus is not seasonal, some scientists are concerned that perhaps the virus may still be at large in China. Because China had been embarrassed by the mishandling of the epidemic, officials there are understandably eager to prove to the world that they can contain the disease. Some have speculated, for example, that in an effort to keep the numbers of SARS victims down, Chinese health officials may have stopped reporting likely SARS cases to WHO.

Another worry is the fact that in May 2003 scientists in China discovered the presence of the SARS virus in a wider variety of animals in food markets in Guangdong Province than previously reported. Originally, SARS was thought to be present in the long-tailed civet cats and rats being sold in food stalls. However, the new findings showed that the virus was also present in raccoon dogs, snakes, wild pigs, bats, badgers, and monkeys being sold as food in the same stalls.

The reaction of WHO officials was one of surprise, because most viruses do not infect such a broad range of animals. "I'm a bit astounded," said one researcher at WHO. "If this virus is present in

*Scientists discovered that the wild pigs, dogs, snakes, and other animals sold as food in Guangdong's markets and restaurants like this one were infected with SARS.*

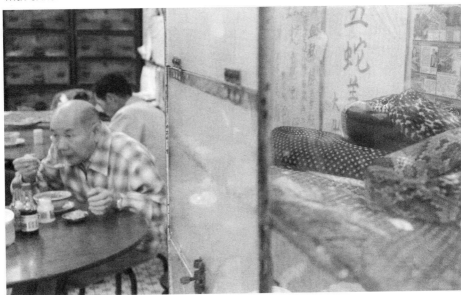

so many species, it would be a big surprise biologically." He went on to admit that if indeed the findings of Chinese researchers were verified, it "would change the ballgame."[78]

## Impossible to Enforce

If it is true that a wider variety of animals carries the virus, it would create a number of new problems. Since it is almost certain that the SARS virus is a crossover from an animal virus, it would mean that there were many carriers of the coronavirus that could possibly infect humans. In that case it is not merely a matter of warning consumers about one or two types of animals, but rather most of the species sold at the markets in southern Guangdong Province. It is believed that the animal virus invades a human host during the handling, slaughtering, or cooking of infected animals. (Researchers do not think that eating animals once they are cooked poses any threat.)

Soon after the link was identified between wild animals and SARS, the Chinese government tried to crack down on the animal markets, banning the sale, capture, transport, or purchase of almost all wild animals—dead or alive. In addition, provincial government officials warned that they would conduct unannounced visits to the markets, restaurants, and ports where the trade in wild animals often occurs. A media campaign began at the same time, urging citizens to "cultivate enlightened and hygienic eating habits, and not eat wild animals."[79]

Yet those who live in southern China say that very little has changed since that time, and animals are as available as ever. In fact, hours after the ban was declared, not only were such animals on sale, but the price had increased, too. For instance, the price of long-tailed civet cats went up from about twenty to more than ninety dollars.

## "It's Fun"

The ban has forced vendors to be more careful not to be caught selling exotic animals, and experts say that usually a raid by health officials or police will not catch many. One reporter was in Guangdong Province when rumors of a raid by government officers circulated, and he was amazed at how quickly the exotic animals dealers disappeared. "One woman placed her turtles into a black trash bag," he writes, "slung it over her shoulder and fled. About twenty more hawkers quickly followed, wheeling cartloads of caged animals with them before vanishing into alleyways and storefronts surrounding the covered market."[80]

Many feel that it will be nearly impossible to enforce the ban, since there is so much money to be made in the markets. They compare the business of selling exotic animals to drug trafficking, insisting that as long as the business is highly profitable, there will always be dealers of such animals. The profits are there because of the demand for such animals, and is not likely to go away.

Many Chinese eat exotic animals because they believe there are health benefits in doing so. The long-tailed civet cat, for example, is believed to boost a person's immune system, while eating various types of snakes is thought to make men more virile. Giant Chinese salamanders are believed to help one's complexion stay smooth. For most of the food market's customers, however, the biggest draw is the experience of eating something different. "It's fun," admits one. "You point to an item on the menu and ask your friends, have you eaten that? No? Well, I have."[81]

Such strong resistance of many Chinese to changing their eating habits has led some scientists to search for ways to lessen the danger of animal-to-human transmission of viruses such as SARS. One University of Hong Kong microbiologist has suggested that long-tailed civet cats be raised on farms, where they could be tested for disease on a regular basis. The slaughterhouses, too, could be controlled by health agencies so that they met approved standards for hygiene and sanitation. Until the sale and slaughter of wild animals is taken out of the hands of individuals, however, the presence of viruses will always be a threat.

## SARS and Developing Nations

Another ongoing worry among international health officials is that if SARS does recur, its effect in developing countries will be

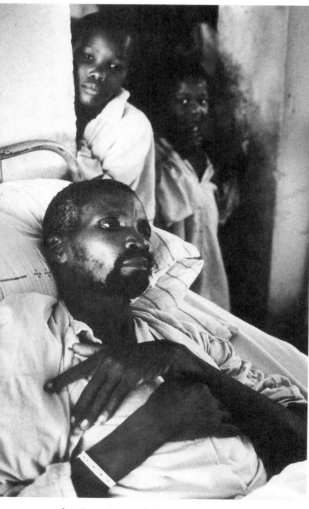

*Should the SARS epidemic recur, it could be devastating to AIDS patients like this African man, and to others with severely weakened immune systems.*

frightening. Scientists know that patients whose immune systems were already weakened from other conditions were more likely to die from SARS. In fact, more than two-thirds of the deaths in every age category were people suffering from chronic diseases. For many people in developing nations, chronic disease is a way of life.

That means that the more than 30 million HIV-infected Africans are especially at risk. Most AIDS patients in South Africa, which has the highest incidence of the disease, do not get treatment, since the majority of sufferers are poor. State hospitals are overwhelmed with the numbers of people needing care, and often must turn people away. "We are already living a nightmare here," says one South African doctor. "Six hundred people are dying each day from AIDS in South Africa, but if SARS comes into a community, it may be as bad as the 1918 influenza epidemic."[82]

Worried about the potential for a devastating epidemic in South Africa, the government has set up a twenty-four-hour clinic at the Cape Town Airport so that international travelers can be checked for symptoms of SARS. Each plane arriving at the airport from a SARS-affected country must be boarded by a public health official, who hands out information about SARS and phone numbers to call if a person suspects he or she may be ill.

Although many hail the government's response to SARS as helpful, others say that the biggest danger is not from international travelers but the millions of poor South Africans who have no access to health care or information about the disease. "People now know about SARS, they are worried about the symptoms and those who fly here with the disease will let medical people know immediately once they feel sick," says one South African specialist. "But what about their gardener or maid, who lives in the township [where the poorest segment of the population lives], and goes home that night with a cough?"[83]

## Ripe for an Epidemic

South Africa is one of many places on the planet where impoverished people could be decimated by SARS. Many researchers at WHO were nervous about the consequences of an outbreak in India, whose 1 billion people live in the most crowded of conditions. Since scientists believe that the outbreak in Hong Kong's Amoy Gardens housing complex was caused by feces of a person with SARS, the likelihood of a major outbreak in India—where only one-fourth of the citizens have toilets—is very strong.

Many nations of the world are also hampered by impoverished, almost nonexistent health care systems. In India, for example, most people have no health insurance, so sick people often wait a long time before going to the doctor. And doctors are scarce—in 2000 it was estimated that in India there were only five doctors for every thousand people, and only one small health center for every eighty thousand people. "The danger is extremely great," says one Indian university professor. "Over time the health system has become weaker and weaker."[84]

Some health care systems are so impoverished that they lack even the basics necessary to treat someone with SARS—or any other contagious disease. Kenya, which is one of the better-equipped African nations, has only ten respirators in the entire country. The Philippines, which spends only 2 percent of its annual budget on its citizens' health, cannot even afford to buy

*Experts fear that a SARS outbreak in poor countries like India and the Philippines would be catastrophic. Most citizens of such countries cannot even afford the basic protection of surgical masks.*

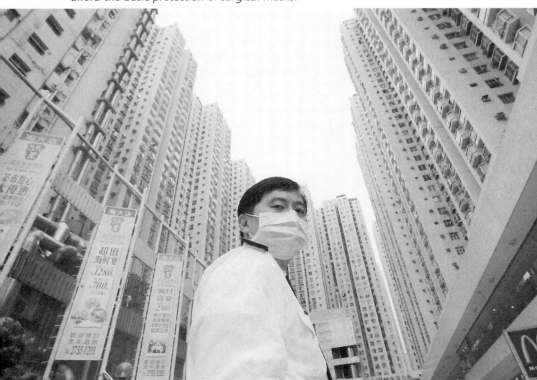

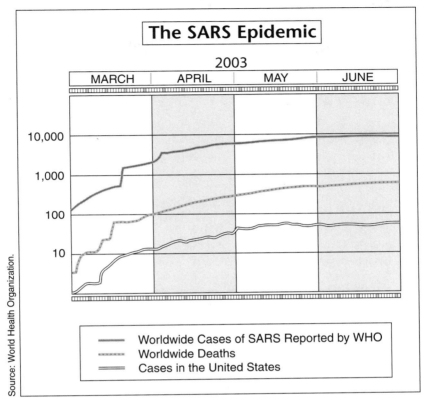

**The SARS Epidemic**

2003

| MARCH | APRIL | MAY | JUNE |

- ——— Worldwide Cases of SARS Reported by WHO
- ·······  Worldwide Deaths
- ════ Cases in the United States

Source: World Health Organization.

gloves and masks for its emergency room technicians. Few disagree that SARS—or any contagious respiratory disease—could kill thousands, or tens of thousands, in such countries before it was through.

## Learning Lessons

One of the most important aspects of the SARS crisis is that it has shown the weaknesses in the health care systems around the world. If the disease returns, as many researchers believe it will, it is important that governments and health agencies learn from the mistakes that were made during the 2003 outbreak of the disease.

For one thing, it is clear that honest, prompt, accurate reporting of the disease is vital to containing it. China's coverup of its first cases directly led to the worldwide spread of SARS. Barry R. Bloom, the dean of the Harvard School of Public Health, says that it is pointless for any nation to use deception when it comes to a virus like SARS. "In infectious diseases, it helps no one to either deny you have a problem, or to be dishonest in reporting it," he says, "because if you do, and you do have spread, you are going to get caught."[85]

But inaccuracy can be just as devasting as deceit, and China is only one of several nations where botched diagnoses allowed SARS-infected patients to spread the disease. In Toronto, an investigation of health officials' handling of the SARS crisis there found a lengthy list of mistakes that worsened the city's epidemic. One of the most flagrant errors was the misdiagnosis of patients. Although many exhibited symptoms of the virus, doctors sent them back into the community, assuring relatives that the patients did not have SARS. As a result, relatives and health care workers became infected.

## "It's the Dumbest Thing in the World"

Toronto's health officials say that one lesson they learned from their experience with SARS was the woeful state of their patient-tracking system. As Toronto's outbreak worsened in April and May, the public health system was overwhelmed by the task of keeping track of thousands of people who had been exposed to the virus and were at risk of developing SARS, as well as the many people in quarantine.

Because of underfunding, the public health office had to rely on a paper-based tracking system—far more time-consuming and prone to errors than a computer-based one. The tracking system was so inaccurate, for example, that some people who were at risk for developing SARS were never called and warned, while others were called several times. Two families were not called until after their relatives had died of SARS.

One health official defends her office, saying that they worked as hard as they could with an antiquated system. She describes how hard it was to keep track of so many individuals:

> Someone takes the file. Where is the file? Okay, well, you look that way and I will look this way. It's the dumbest thing in the world. I can't believe this is the state of affairs. It's amazing to

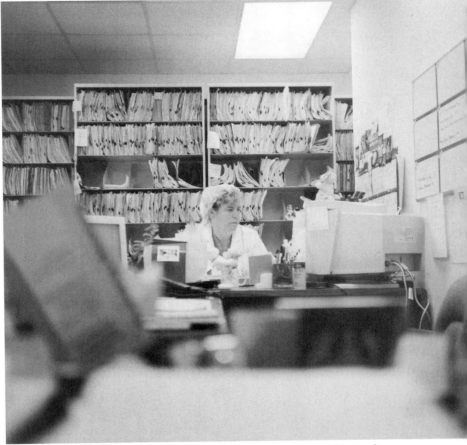

*During the SARS outbreak in Toronto, doctors learned the importance of a computer-based patient tracking system like the one this nurse is using.*

me that we have been able to manage the way we have, given that degree of inadequate support on these central functions with basic technology.[86]

## "The Crossroads of the World"

Another lesson of the SARS crisis was how important a part Hong Kong played in the epidemic, and how vulnerable to disease the region is. Hong Kong lies at the very edge of southern China, a region that is historically where many flu viruses and

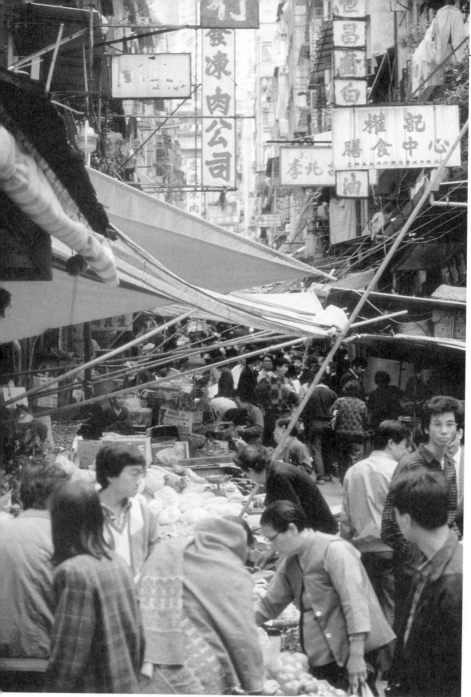

The crowded streets of Hong Kong are breeding grounds for disease. The city's large population, its crowded conditions, and the number of tourists who visit annually make contagious illnesses difficult to control.

other potential epidemics begin. There are an estimated 4 million border crossings from southern China into Hong Kong each month by people who may very well be carrying a number of germs.

Hong Kong is also vulnerable because the crowded, heavily populated conditions in the city make any contagious disease difficult to control. There are many housing projects like the Amoy Gardens, and a broken sewer pipe or a faulty ventilation system could easily spread a virus to hundreds of thousands of people within a few days. Doctors agree that in the SARS epidemic of 2003, Hong Kong was fortunate to keep the number of infections at 1,755 and the death count at 295.

Finally, Hong Kong's role as the busiest air travel hub in all of Asia is another reason the region is such a worry to infectious disease experts. With seventy airlines in operation there, there are almost unlimited opportunities for the virus to spread anywhere on the planet. "Hong Kong is at the crossroads of the world, certainly," says one WHO official. "It's not only susceptible to many diseases coming in, but also to exporting diseases, and they travel around the world."[87]

## Police and Health Officials

WHO officials are convinced that health agencies throughout the world would be wise to see how Hong Kong was able to contain the spread of SARS, given its high vulnerability to contagious diseases. It was successful, say experts, because once Hong Kong's public health department realized the danger, it began a thorough tracking of all personal contacts of each SARS patient who had been seen in a hospital there.

Not only did public health workers do the tracking, but police officers helped, too. All family members or friends who had been in contact with a person infected with SARS were found and confined to their homes. Some worried that this zealous tracking partnership might be an infringement of civil liberties, but most health care workers in Hong Kong and elsewhere were pleased with the system—and other nations have taken note. "I'm convinced that the way that the health authorities, the Department of Health and the police department have begun to work together on this outbreak will not only be copied in future outbreaks here in Hong Kong, but in cases throughout the world," said one WHO official, "because it's a very important marriage of databases."[88]

## Is the World Ready?

Hong Kong is not the only place where strategies have been mapped out in the event that SARS returns. In the United States, where only a handful of confirmed cases were verified, health officials have taken inventory in various cities, making certain that there are enough respirators and other tools needed to care for victims. Many experts say that even before the SARS outbreak worldwide, the United States was already fairly organized for a large outbreak of some infectious disease. The terrorist attacks of September 11, 2001, had alerted the nation that its procedures for a bioterrorist attack needed to be shored up.

The anthrax scare, as well as the heightened nervousness about the use of the smallpox virus as a weapon, created an urgency throughout the medical community. As a result, communications between hospitals and public health authorities have been in a constant process of improvement, and readiness is the number one priority. Hospitals need to be equipped to handle "surge capacity," which is the sudden influx of hundreds of new patients at one time. By 2004 city hospitals are expected to be ready to handle as many as fifteen hundred emergency patients in a single day.

In the United States, many doctors and public health officials have been impressed with the sense of cooperation between hospitals—which often compete for business. Emergency rooms at various hospitals have begun cross-credentialing patient information so doctors have access to information about patients no matter at what facility they receive care. The cooperation has saved hospitals money on supplies, too. "We're talking about buying [supplies] in bulk, in economies of scale," says one Dallas physician, "with everybody participating. Everybody is anteing up."[89]

## New Tools to Fight SARS

If or when SARS does make a comeback, scientists are banking on new tools with which to fight it. Although experts predict a vaccine will not be available until at least 2006, there are other things that could be valuable in saving lives. One would be an accurate test for SARS. Tests at the current time are not accurate unless a patient has been infected for at least twelve days. In that time, that patient will have infected dozens of other people.

However, in July 2003 one Swiss drugmaker announced that it had developed a test that could diagnose even a tiny trace of the virus in a patient's bloodstream. Although the product first needs to be clinically assessed, doctors say that such a test would be extremely good news. Another test being developed by the Public Health Research Institute is rapid, too. It uses tiny beacons of DNA with a light-emitting molecule at one end. When

*Doctors are working to develop a vaccine against SARS and are researching the use of antibodies to help infected patients fight the disease.*

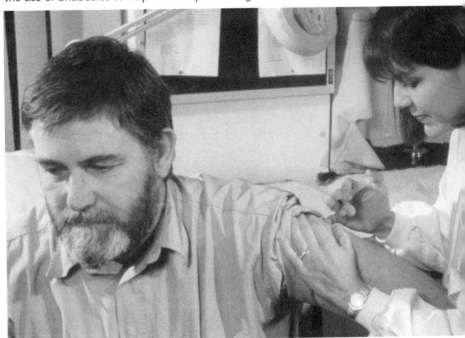

the beacon senses a bit of the genetic makeup of the virus, the molecular light flashes.

As yet, there is not a surefire drug to cure SARS, but some progress has been made. Doctors know, for example, that a combination of the antiviral drug Ribavirin combined with an AIDS drug called Kaletra has great promise. Ribavirin tries to damage the virus, while Kaletra cuts the virus's ability to replicate itself. Doctors in Hong Kong have said that they will use a combination of the drugs if SARS returns. However, some doctors are less enthusiastic. They point out that there is a risk to using the drugs, for they may cause red blood cells to break down, and in some patients, that would ultimately interfere with the body's ability to fight off disease.

One very promising study by the University of Massachusetts Medical School is looking at producing antibodies, which are normally made by the body as it fights an infection. If antibodies could be produced in a laboratory, there might be a way to give an injection to a patient to fight SARS, or to healthy people to prevent it. The director of the study says she is optimistic that such a vaccine is possible. "We're pretty convinced," she says, "that if you give the right antibody to the right folks at the right time, you can be pretty effective in shutting down an outbreak."[90]

## Looking Ahead

Though such promising improvements are reason for medical authorities to be hopeful, they know that SARS may very well reappear before drugs or tests are completed. If there is another outbreak, doctors fervently hope that it occurs within a pool of people that has access to good medical care. With prompt, accurate reporting, experts believe that they can halt the spread of SARS before it becomes an epidemic—again.

# Notes

### Introduction: The Faces of SARS

1. Quoted in James Kelly, "Making News on the SARS Front," *Time*, May 5, 2003, p. 8.
2. Quoted in Claudia Kalb, "The Mystery of SARS," *Newsweek*, May 5, 2003, p. 29.
3. Quoted in Kalb, "The Mystery of SARS," p. 28.
4. Lily, telephone interview by author, September 18, 2003.

### Chapter 1: The Secret Killer

5. Quoted in BBC News, "Eyewitness: Vietnam's SARS Survivor," April 17, 2003. www.news.bbc.co.uk.
6. Quoted in BBC News, "Eyewitness."
7. Quoted in Peter Wonacott, Susan V. Lawrence, and David Murphy, "China Faces Up to SARS Criticism," *Wall Street Journal*, April 3, 2003, p. A13.
8. Quoted in Elizabeth Rosenthal, "From China's Provinces, a Crafty Germ Spreads," *New York Times*, April 27, 2003, p. A3.
9. Rosenthal, "From China's Provinces," p. A3.
10. Quoted in Donald McNeil Jr., "Rise of a Virus: The Global Response," *New York Times*, May 4, 2003, p. 1.
11. Quoted in Steven Frank, "Tale of Two Countries: Canada," *Time*, May 5, 2003, p. 56.
12. Quoted in Frank, "Tale of Two Countries: Canada," p. 57.
13. Quoted in McNeil, "Rise of a Virus," p. 1.
14. Hannah Beech, "How Bad Is It?" *Time International*, May 5, 2003, p. 12.
15. Quoted in Rosenthal, "From China's Provinces," p. A3.
16. Quoted in Leslie Chang, "In South China, Mix of Old and

New Helps Spawn Virus," *Wall Street Journal*, April 2, 2003, p. A1.

17. Quoted in Leslie Chang, "In South China," p. A1.

18. Quoted in Romesh Ratnesar and Hannah Beech, "Tale of Two Countries: China," *Time*, May 5, 2003, p. 55.

19. Hannah Beech, "Regional Affair," *Time International*, April 28, 2003, p. 10.

20. Beech, "Regional Affair," p. 10.

21. Quoted in Hannah Beech, "Unmasking a Crisis," *Time International*, April 21, 2003, p. 40.

22. Quoted in Beech, "Unmasking a Crisis," p. 40.

23. Quoted in Hannah Beech, "Doing Battle with the Bug," *Time International*, April 14, 2003, p. 44.

## Chapter 2: Investigating SARS

24. Quoted in Claudia Kalb, "Tracking SARS," *Newsweek*, April 28, 2003, p. 36.

25. Quoted in Leslie Chang, "In South China," p. A1.

26. Quoted in *Wall Street Journal*, "Labs Collaborate World-Wide to Identify Deadly Virus," March 26, 2003, p. B1.

27. Quoted in Kalb, "Tracking SARS," p. 36.

28. Quoted in Kalb, "Tracking SARS," p. 36.

29. Michael Lemonick, "Will SARS Strike Here?" *Time*, April 14, 2003, p. 72.

30. Quoted in Denise Grady and Lawrence Altman, "Rise of a Virus: Cracking the Mystery," *New York Times*, May 26, 2003, p. A1.

31. Quoted in Grady and Altman, "Rise of a Virus," p. A1.

32. Quoted in Grady and Altman, "Rise of a Virus," p. A1.

33. Quoted in Kalb, "The Mystery of SARS," p. 28.

34. Sita Li, interview by author, Minneapolis, Minnesota, August 12, 2003.

35. Rosenthal, "From China's Provinces," p. A3.

36. Quoted in Lemonick, "Will SARS Strike Here?" p. 72.

37. Quoted in Lemonick, "Will SARS Strike Here?" p. 72.

38. Quoted in Lemonick, "Will SARS Strike Here?" p. 72.

## Chapter 3: Life with SARS

39. Kathy Chen, "China Is As Good at Fighting SARS As at Hiding It," *Wall Street Journal*, June 4, 2003, p. D3.
40. Quoted in Rosenthal, "From China's Provinces," p. A3.
41. Quoted in Rosenthal, "From China's Provinces," p. A3.
42. Quoted in Amanda Gardner, "Life 'Surreal' for Nurse Under SARS Quarantine," *HealthDayNews*, Healthfinder, May 30, 2003. www.healthfinder.gov.
43. Quoted in Gardner, "Life 'Surreal.'"
44. Quoted in Beech, "Doing Battle with the Bug," p. 44.
45. Quoted in Associated Press, "Chinese Trash Building over SARS Quarantine," *HoustonChronicle.com*, May 5, 2003. www.chron.com.
46. Melissa Hinebauch, "Breathing Easy—Until We Go Home Again," *Newsweek*, May 12, 2003, p. 20.
47. Quoted in Matt Pottinger and Rebecca Buckman, "Holding Their Breath," *Wall Street Journal*, March 28, 2003, p. A1.
48. Quoted in Steve Friess, "Questions Escalating with the Deadly Epidemic," *USA Today*, April 7, 2003, p. D9.
49. Quoted in Lawrence Altman, "Behind the Mask, the Fear of SARS," *New York Times*, June 24, 2003, p. F1.
50. Quoted in Altman, "Behind the Mask," p. F1.
51. Quoted in Altman, "Behind the Mask," p. F1.
52. Quoted in Geoffrey Fowler, "In China, SARS Robs Families of Chance to Say Goodbye," *Wall Street Journal*, May 30, 2003, p. A1.
53. Quoted in Fowler, "In China, SARS Robs Families," p. A1.
54. Quoted in Fowler, "In China, SARS Robs Families," p. A1.
55. Quoted in Kelly, "Making News on the SARS Front," p. 8.
56. Quoted in Kelly, "Making News on the SARS Front," p. 8.
57. Quoted in Altman, "Behind the Mask," p. F1.

## Chapter 4: SARS, Politics, and the Economy

58. Quoted in Beech, "Unmasking a Crisis," p. 40.
59. Quoted in Beech, "How Bad Is It?" p. 12.
60. Quoted in Ratnesar and Beech, "A Tale of Two Countries: China," p. 54.

61. Quoted in Beech, "Regional Affair," p. 10.

62. Quoted in Gordon Chang, "SARS Crisis: New Disease, New Leaders, Same Old Regime," *China Brief,* Jamestown Foundation, April 22, 2003.

63. Quoted in Ratnesar and Beech, "A Tale of Two Countries: China," p. 54.

64. Quoted in Gordon Chang, "SARS Crisis: New Disease."

65. Quoted in Willy Lam, "SARS Crisis: Beijing's Leadership Slowly Responds," *China Brief,* Jamestown Foundation, April 22, 2003.

66. Quoted in Ratnesar and Beech, "A Tale of Two Countries: China," p. 54.

67. Quoted in Beech, "How Bad Is It?" p. 12.

68. Quoted in Beech, "How Bad Is It?" p. 12.

69. Quoted in Keith Bradsher, "Economies Sickened by a Virus, and Fear," *New York Times,* April 21, 2003, p. A1.

70. Keith Bradsher, "Hong Kong Tourism Battered by Outbreak," *New York Times,* April 13, 2003.

71. Quoted in Bradsher, "Economies Sickened," p. A1.

72. Quoted in Bradsher, "Economies Sickened," p. A1.

73. Quoted in Kalb, "The Mystery of SARS," p. 28.

74. Quoted in Clifford Krauss, "SARS Abates in Toronto, but Tourism Still Lags," *New York Times,* July 26, 2003.

75. Quoted in Associated Press, "Precautionary Procedures," SI.com, April 23, 2003. www.sportsillustrated.cnn.com.

**Chapter 5: SARS and the Future**

76. Quoted in Brad Wright, "Experts: SARS Comeback Likely Next Winter," CNN.com, May 21, 2003. www.cnn.com.

77. Quoted in Keith Bradsher, "SARS Declared Contained, with No Cases in Past 20 Days," *New York Times,* July 6, 2003.

78. Quoted in Lawrence Altman, "The SARS Enigma," *New York Times,* June 8, 2003.

79. Quoted in Matt Pottinger, "In Shenzhou, China, Wild Animal Market Eludes a Crackdown," *Wall Street Journal,* May 28, 2003, p. A1.

80. Pottinger, "In Shenzhou, China," p. A1.

81. Quoted in Pottinger, "In Shenzhou, China," p. A1.

82. Quoted in *Newsweek International*, "Waiting for Disaster," May 12, 2003, p. 28.

83. Quoted in *Newsweek International*, "Waiting for Disaster," p. 28.

84. Quoted in *Newsweek International*, "Waiting for Disaster," p. 28.

85. Quoted in Keith Bradsher, "Isolation, an Old Medical Tool, Has SARS Fading," *New York Times*, June 21, 2003, p. A1.

86. Quoted in Keith Donovan and Tanya Talaga, "SARS: The Chain of Errors," *Toronto Star*, September 20, 2003. www.thestar.com.

87. Quoted in Bradsher, "Isolation," p. A1.

88. Quoted in Bradsher, "Isolation," p. A1.

89. Quoted in Sheryl Gay Stolberg and Judith Miller, "Threats and Responses: Many Worry That Nation Is Still Highly Vulnerable to Germ Attack," *New York Times*, September 9, 2002, p. A16.

90. Quoted in Marilyn Chase and Antonio Regalado, "Search Continues for SARS Drugs," *Wall Street Journal*, September 17, 2003, p. A7.

# *Organizations to Contact*

**Centers for Disease Control and Prevention (CDC)**
1600 Clifton Rd., Atlanta, GA 30333
(404) 639-3311
www.cdc.gov

The CDC's goal is to promote health and quality of life by preventing and controlling disease. The organization has developed vital partnerships with public and private medical groups that can provide information and assistance to people in the United States and throughout the world. One of the CDC's functions is to investigate outbreaks of new and dangerous diseases such as SARS.

**National Institutes of Health (NIH)**
9000 Rockville Pike, Bethesda, MD 20892
www.nih.gov

This organization is one of the most sophisticated medical research centers in the world. Comprising twenty-seven separate institutes and centers, the NIH is dedicated to acquiring new knowledge to help prevent, detect, diagnose, and treat diseases, as well as to support education about them.

**World Health Organization (WHO)**
Avenue Appia 20, 1211 Geneva 27, Switzerland
www.who.int

A part of the United Nations, the WHO works to help people achieve physical, mental, and social well-being. The WHO's website contains up-to-date information on diseases affecting people all over the world.

# For Further Reading

## Books

Margrete Lamond, *Plague and Pestilence: Deadly Diseases That Changed the World*. Chicago: Allen & Unwin, 1997. Excellent examples of the way people have reacted to sudden, contagious diseases. Good index.

P.C. Leung and E.E. Ooi, eds., *SARS War: Combating the Disease*. Singapore: World Scientific, 2003. Although much of the material is incomplete, the book does contain some helpful information on the history of emerging diseases in China.

Elinor Levy, *The New Killer Diseases: How the Alarming Evolution of Mutant Germs Threatens Us All*. New York: Crown, 2003. Excellent section on the mutation of viruses, though challenging reading.

Fred Ramen, *Influenza*. New York: Rosen, 2001. Very good section on the 1918 epidemic, to which SARS researchers refer as the nightmare of contagious diseases. Helpful index.

## Websites

**CDC** (www.cdc.gov). This is the official site of the Centers for Disease Control and Prevention, and it contains a wealth of information about SARS, its spread, and what is being done to combat it.

**World Health Organization** (www.who.int). This site has up-to-the-minute articles and bulletins about any SARS news from around the world, including travel warnings about the virus or any other communicable disease.

# Works Consulted

**Periodicals**

Lawrence Altman, "Behind the Mask, the Fear of SARS," *New York Times*, June 24, 2003.

——, "The SARS Enigma," *New York Times*, June 8, 2003.

Hannah Beech, "Doing Battle with the Bug," *Time International*, April 14, 2003.

——, "How Bad Is It?" *Time International*, May 5, 2003.

——, "Regional Affair," *Time International*, April 28, 2003.

——, "Unmasking a Crisis," *Time International*, April 21, 2003.

Keith Bradsher, "Economies Sickened by a Virus, and Fear," *New York Times*, April 21, 2003.

——, "Hong Kong Tourism Battered by Outbreak," *"New York Times*, April 13, 2003.

——, "Isolation, an Old Medical Tool, Has SARS Fading," *New York Times*, June 21, 2003.

——, "SARS Declared Contained, with No Cases in Past 20 Days," *New York Times*, July 6, 2003.

Gordon Chang, "SARS Crisis: New Disease, New Leaders, Same Old Regime," *China Brief*, Jamestown Foundation, April 22, 2003.

Leslie Chang, "In South China, Mix of Old and New Helps Spawn Virus," *Wall Street Journal*, April 2, 2003.

Marilyn Chase and Antonio Regalado, "Search Continues for SARS Drugs," *Wall Street Journal*, September 17, 2003.

Kathy Chen, "China Is As Good at Fighting SARS As at Hiding It," *Wall Street Journal*, June 4, 2003.

Geoffrey Fowler, "In China, SARS Robs Families of Chance to Say Goodbye," *Wall Street Journal*, May 30, 2003.

Geoffrey Fowler and Ben Dolven, "If SARS Stages a Comeback, Is the World Ready?" *Wall Street Journal*, August 14, 2003.

Steven Frank, "Tale of Two Countries: Canada," *Time*, May 5, 2003.

Steve Friess, "Questions Escalating with the Deadly Epidemic," *USA Today*, April 7, 2003.

Denise Grady and Lawrence Altman, "Rise of a Virus: Cracking the Mystery," *New York Times*, May 26, 2003.

Melissa Hinebauch, "Breathing Easy—Until We Go Home Again," *Newsweek*, May 12, 2003.

Claudia Kalb, "The Mystery of SARS," *Newsweek*, May 5, 2003.

———, "Tracking SARS," *Newsweek*, April 28, 2003.

James Kelly, "Making News on the SARS Front," *Time*, May 5, 2003.

Clifford Krauss, "SARS Abates in Toronto, but Tourism Still Lags," *New York Times*, July 26, 2003.

Willy Lam, "SARS Crisis: Beijing's Leadership Slowly Responds," *China Brief*, Jamestown Foundation, April 22, 2003.

Michael Lemonick, "Will SARS Strike Here? "*Time*, April 14, 2003.

Donald McNeil Jr., "Rise of a Virus: The Global Response," *New York Times*, May 4, 2003.

*Newsweek International*, "Waiting for Disaster," May 12, 2003.

Matt Pottinger, "In Shenzhou, China, Wild Animal Market Eludes a Crackdown," *Wall Street Journal*, May 28, 2003.

Matt Pottinger and Rebecca Buckman, "Holding Their Breath," *Wall Street Journal*, March 28, 2003.

Romesh Ratnesar and Hannah Beech, "Tale of Two Countries: China," *Time*, May 5, 2003.

Elizabeth Rosenthal, "From China's Provinces, a Crafty Germ Spreads," "*New York Times*, April 27, 2003.

Sheryl Gay Stolberg and Judith Miller, "Threats and Responses: Many Worry That Nation Is Still Highly Vulnerable to Germ Attack," *New York Times*, September 9, 2002.

*Wall Street Journal*, "Labs Collaborate World-Wide to Identify Deadly Virus," March 26, 2003.

Peter Wonacott, Susan V. Lawrence, and David Murphy, "China Faces Up to SARS Criticism," *Wall Street Journal*, April 3, 2003.

## Internet Sources

Associated Press, "Chinese Trash Building over SARS Quarantine," *HoustonChronicle.com*, May 5, 2003. www.chron.com.

————, "Precautionary Procedures," SI.com, April 23, 2003. www.sportsillustrated.cnn.com.

BBC News, "Eyewitness: Vietnam's SARS Survivor," April 17, 2003. www.news.bbc.co.uk.

Keith Donovan and Tanya Talaga, "SARS: The Chain of Errors," *Toronto Star*, September 20, 2003. www.thestar.com.

Amanda Gardner, "Life 'Surreal' for Nurse Under SARS Quarantine," *Health Day News*, Healthfinder, May 30, 2003. www.healthfinder.gov.

Brad Wright, "Experts: SARS Comeback Likely Next Winter," CNN.com, May 21, 2003. www.cnn.com.

# Index

AIDS, 28, 32, 36, 43, 90
  in China, 60
  in South Africa, 80–81
air travel, 10–11, 20, 28, 45–46,
  68, 70–73
ambulances, patients hidden in,
  25
Amoy Gardens, 41, 48, 59, 81, 87
animals, 31, 34–35, 37–39, 77–79
anthrax, 18, 88
antibiotics, 13, 15, 18–19, 32
  *see also* drugs
antibodies, 38, 90
appetite, loss of, 13
Asia
  effects on, 68–69, 71, 73
  spread in, 30, 48–49, 57
asthma, 43
Australia, 71–72
autopsies, 30

bacteria, 31–32
baseball. *See* Toronto Blue Jays
Beijing (China), 23–25, 63–65, 67
bioterrorism, 12, 18, 88
bird flu, 31
  *see also* flu
blood samples, 29–31, 33
blood tests, 38
breathing, difficulty in, 13, 15,
  20
Building 15 (CDC), 30–31

business, 51, 68, 71, 73
  *see also* economy

Canada, 19–20, 46–48, 52–53,
  73–74
  *see also* Toronto
cancer, 43
Cape Town Airport, 81
Cathay Pacific Airlines, 71
cells, 32, 37
Centers for Disease Control
  (CDC), 11, 18–19, 23, 29–31,
  33–34
  *see also* World Health
    Organization
Chan, Henry Likyuen, 10
children, 49–54
China
  effects on, 11, 24, 54, 67–71
  government cover-up in,
    15–16, 18–20, 22–26, 60–66,
    77, 83–84
  health care workers in, 52,
    62–63
  origins of SARS in, 10, 13–15,
    31, 76–77, 85–87
  political system of, 44, 62–67
  preventive measures in, 44–45,
    48–51, 66–67, 77–79
  spread of SARS in, 14–18
  *see also* Hong Kong
China-Japan Friendship
  Hospital, 25

cholera, 28
church attendance, 56–57
civit cats, 38, 77–79
 *see also* animals
clothing, protective, 18–20, 45,
 47, 52
colds, 34, 76
 *see also* flu; pneumonia
Communist Party, 62, 65, 67
coronaviruses, 34–38, 76, 78
 *see also* viruses
coughing
 as symptom, 10, 13–14, 20, 38
 transmission by, 26, 39, 42
crisis team (WHO), 31–33, 37
cures, 42, 90
 *see also* antibiotics

Dawson, Peggy, 47–48
death rituals, 54–56
deaths
 from AIDS, 28
 from 1918 influenza, 29
 from SARS, 10, 18–20, 49, 58,
 80, 87
developing countries, 79–81
discrimination, 59
diseases, contagious, 12, 28–29,
 31, 87
disinfectant, 44–45
DNA microarray, 34–35
DNA tests, 89–90
doctors. *See* health care workers
drugs, 42–43, 90

Ebola, 28, 36
economy, 11, 15, 24, 51, 67–73
epidemics, 28, 77, 80–81
 SARS as, 22–25, 44, 47–48,
 67–69, 84, 90
epidemiologists, 31, 33
exposure, 46–48
face masks. *See* masks,

protective
family members
 psychological effects on, 11,
 54–58, 62–63
 quarantine of, 46, 87
 rate of infection among, 65, 84
 *see also* victims
fatigue, 14, 19, 38–39
feces, 41, 81
fever, 10, 13–14, 19–20, 38, 42
flu, 34
 origins of, in China, 31, 85–87
 SARS mistaken for, 13–14, 18,
 38, 84
 *see also* influenza epidemic
folk remedies, 18
food stalls, 38, 77–79
funerals, 56

genetics. *See* viruses, genetic
 makeup of
germs, 30, 38, 44, 51
global alerts, 20, 31, 67, 70, 74
Guangdong Province (China)
 government cover-up in,
 15–16
 origins in, 13–15, 22, 28, 38,
 77–79
 spread in, 17–19, 67
 *see also* Hong Kong
Guangzhou (China), 17

hand washing, 44
Hanoi (Vietnam), 19–21, 29
 *see also* Vietnam
headaches, 13
health care systems, weaknesses
 of, 63, 79–85, 88
health care workers, 46–48, 59
 lack of information and, 15–18,
 25–27, 62–63
 rate of infection among, 13–15,
 20–21, 23–24, 29, 52–54, 84

HIV. *See* AIDS
Holmes, Kathryn, 37
Hong Kong
  effects on, 54–59, 67, 69–71
  health care workers in, 52
  preventive measures in, 51,
    87–88, 90
  spread in, 10–11, 19–20, 26–27,
    40–42, 48, 81, 85–87
hospitals, 20–21, 23–25, 47, 88
housing projects, 87
  *see also* Amoy Gardens
Hu Jintao, 65–67
human contact, 26–27, 51

immunity, 42
incubation period, 46, 89
India, 81–82
infection. *See* SARS,
  transmission of; *specific types of
  transmission*
influenza epidemic (1918), 29,
  81
information, lack of, 15–18, 20
insomnia, 15
insulin, 37
Internet, 15–16, 18, 23, 28, 33
Iraq war, 33, 72
isolation, 17–21, 23–24, 38
  *see also* quarantine

Jiang Zemin, 67
joints, aching, 13–15

Kaletra, 90
Kenya, 82

laboratory research. *See* research
  efforts
Lastman, Mel, 74
life, daily, effects on, 44–59
  *see also* society
Liu Jianlun, 19–20

livestock, 31, 34
  *see also* animals
lungs, 15, 39
lung tissue, 30–31

malaria, 28
masks, protective, 14, 18–20,
  44–47, 51–54, 63, 71
media
  Chinese, 15, 44, 62–63, 78
  international, 58, 66
medicine. *See* antibiotics; drugs
microbiologists, 33
microscopes, 32, 34
mistakes, in handling of SARS,
  83–84
monkeys, kidney cells of, 33
  *see also* animals
muscles, aching, 13–14
mutations, of viruses, 12, 31,
  37–38
  *see also* viruses

North York General Hospital,
  47
Number 2 People's Hospital,
  17–18
nurses. *See* health care workers

panic, 18, 22, 67
pathogens, 30, 34
patient-tracking systems, 84–85,
  87–88
Peking University People's
  Hospital, 23–24
Perl, Trish, 52–54
Philippines, 82–83
phlegm, 14, 42
pigs, 31, 77
  *see also* animals
pneumonia, 13, 15–16, 28, 34
politics, 60–67
poor people, susceptibility
  among, 80–83

prevention. *See* SARS,
   prevention of; *specific types of
   prevention*
protein spikes, 34, 37
Public Health Research
   Institute, 89–90

quarantine, 27, 45–49, 52, 59, 84,
   87

rats, 38, 77
   *see also* animals
research efforts, 20, 28–43
respirators, 13, 15, 82, 88
Ribavirin, 42, 90
rumors, 16, 18, 22–23, 28
rural areas, spread in, 13, 17, 31,
   63, 81–82

SARS
   causes of, 27, 31, 34, 37, 39, 78
   prevention of, 38, 42–54,
      66–67, 77–79, 87–90
   rapid spread of, 10–23, 27–28,
      48, 67, 81–82, 85–87
   recurrence of, 76–77, 79–84,
      88–90
   symptoms of, 10, 13–15, 19–20
   transmission of, 26–27, 37–42,
      52, 56, 77–79
Saudi Arabia, 46
scanning, of air travelers, 45–46
Scarborough Grace Hospital,
   20–21, 47
school, cancellation of, 49
severe acute respiratory
   syndrome. *See* SARS
Shanghai (China), 24–25, 62–63,
   67
Singapore, 19, 21, 45–46, 49–51,
   57
smallpox, 88
sneezing, 26, 39

society, 11–12, 26, 44–59
South Africa, 80–81
sputum, 31
steroids, 42, 58
Stohr, Klaus, 33
superspreaders, 41–42
surgical masks. *See* masks,
   protective
survivors, 58–59
   *see also* victims
symptoms. *See* SARS,
   symptoms of; *specific types of
   symptoms*

Taipei International Spring
   Show, 68
Tan Tock Seng Hospital, 21
temperatures, taking of, 44, 46,
   49
Thailand, 46
Thompson, Tommy, 23
throat tissue, 33–34
Tiananmen Square, protests in,
   67
tissue samples, 19, 29–31, 33
Toronto (Canada)
   effects on, 73–74
   health care workers in, 52–54,
      84
   spread in, 10–12, 20, 27, 31
Toronto Blue Jays (baseball
   team), 74–75
touching, 40, 49, 51
tourism, 11, 68, 74
   *see also* air travel
transmission. *See* SARS,
   transmission of; *specific types of
   transmission*
transportation, 44–45, 49
travel. *See* air travel
treatment. *See* antibiotics; SARS,
   prevention of
trickle-down effect, 68–69

unemployment, 11, 68–69, 71
United States, 52, 72–73, 88
University of California, San
   Francisco, 34
University of Massachusetts
   Medical School, 90

vaccines, 42, 89–90
Vero cells, 33–34
victims, 10–11, 19–20, 54–57, 63,
   65, 84
   *see also* health care workers;
      survivors
Vietnam, 19–21, 29, 52
virology, 36
viruses, 12, 32
   animals as transmitters of, 31,

33–34, 77–79
   genetic makeup of, 34–35,
      37–38, 90
   SARS, 37–40

West Nile disease, 36
World Health Organization
   (WHO), 13, 18–19, 22–25, 66,
   76–78, 87
   global alerts from, 20, 67, 70, 74
   research by, 28–29, 31–34, 37
Wu Yi, 66

Yang Jie, 44–45

Zhejiang Province (China),
   48–49

# Picture Credits

Cover photo: Getty Images
© AFP/CORBIS, 14, 22, 26, 36, 64, 82
AP/Wide World Photos, 55
© Morton Beebe/CORBIS, 86
Mike Cassese/Landov, 11
CDC/James Gathany/Photo Researchers, 61
Kin Cheung/Reuters/Landov, 50, 57
Christine Chew/UPI/Landov, 73
Claro Cortes IV/Reuters/Landov, 16, 72
© Ric Ergenbright/CORBIS, 30
Getty Images, 58
Paul Hilton/EPA/Landov, 77
© So Hing-Keung/CORBIS, 70
Chris Jouan, 69, 83
© Helen King/CORBIS, 85
Russel Knightley/SPL/Photo Researchers, 35
Kyodo/Landov, 53
© Gideon Mendel/CORBIS, 80
Guang Niu/Reuters/Landov, 45, 47
PhotoDisc, 39
Reuters/Landov, 21, 24, 43
© Reuters NewMedia Inc./CORBIS, 32, 40, 54, 66
Geoff Tompkinson/Photo Researchers, 89
Thomas White/Reuters/Landov, 29
Bobby Yip/Landov, 17

## About the Author

Gail B. Stewart received her undergraduate degree from Gustavus Adolphus College in St. Peter, Minnesota. She did her graduate work in English, linguistics, and curriculum study at the College of St. Thomas and the University of Minnesota. She taught English and reading for more than ten years.

She has written over ninety books for young people, including a series for Lucent Books called The Other America. She has written many books on historical topics such as World War I and the Warsaw ghetto.

Stewart and her husband live in Minneapolis with their three sons, Ted, Elliot, and Flynn; two dogs; and a cat. When she is not writing, she enjoys reading, walking, and watching her sons play soccer.